MW01054681

# Medical Astrology
*A Guide to Planetary Pathology*

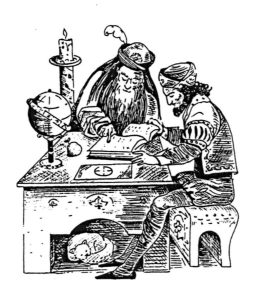

by Judith Hill

# Medical Astrology
## *A Guide to Planetary Pathology*

by Judith Hill

Copyright © 2004 by Judith Hill

All rights reserved.

No part of this book may be reproduced or transmitted in any form or by any means, electronic or mechanical, including photocopying or recording, or by any information storage and retrieval system, without written permission from the author and publisher. Requests may be emailed to: stelliumpress@aol.com

ISBN 1-883376-06-8

*Disclaimer*: the author is not a licensed medical practitioner and is providing astrological opinions only, not medical diagnosis or established medical fact. The author is not advocating the use of astrology as an exclusive or primary medical model or tool. The intent of this book is educational.

Published by Stellium Press, 2005
This book is printed on acid free paper.

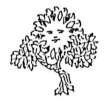

Stellium Press
P.O. Box 86512
Portland, OR 97286
stelliumpress@aol.com

# TABLE OF CONTENTS

*TABLE OF CONTENTS  (continued)*

TABLE OF CONTENTS *(continued)*

ILLUSTRATIONS

# Introduction

Classical Western medical astrology never died as is typically assumed, only later to be resurrected by modern enthusiasts of antiquity. Renegade physicians continued the practice in the West, albeit underground, right on through to our present era. At least three Western doctors of the last century have written excellent texts upon this subject, inclusive of their case studies. In India an extremely close variant has been practiced unabated since the art was introduced.

Medical Astrology escaped the first sanctions of the Church, being considered theologically safe "natural" astrology, and necessary to the study of medicine. Until the sixteenth century, a physician had to pass his exams in this subject. At the University of Bologna, a four year course in Astrology was completed by aspiring physicians of the day. Cecco d'Ascoli, a lecturer at the University of Bologna in the early fourteenth century wrote; "A doctor must of necessity know and take into account the natures of the stars and their conjunctions..."

The medieval theorist Arnals of Villanova, who died in 1313, wrote a book on medical astrology entitled: '*On the Judgments of Sicknesses, According to the Movement of the Planets, for the Not Inconsiderable Assistance of Doctors.*'

There is considerable remnant of astrology's status in medicine from the Greek through the medieval period in our current medical symbols and language. Modern medical textbooks still use our astrologer's symbols for Venus and Mars to indicate "female" and "male". We hear of "venereal" diseases, and varicose "veins", both ailments attributed to Venus; of "lunacy" and the "solar" plexus.

Our literature yet includes reference to "jovial", "mercurial" and "saturnine" temperaments or we might speak of a "martial" man. Even the "menses" is a "moonses", medically acknowledging a link between a woman's monthly cycle and the Moon. And is not the very staff of Mercury (his caduceus), the symbol for the medical profession?

It is even held that the pharmaceutical "rx" sign has an astrological origin because the precise symbol means "radix", an old term for the astrological natal chart. The prescribing physician of the medieval period placed this mark on the client's prescription to indicate "I've seen the horoscope".

However, medical astrology is far older than the medieval period. The doctrine of zodiac sign rulership over parts of the body may date to at least 400 B.C. The Babylonian and Assyrian records have evidence of this tradition. The earliest origins are uncertain, possibly Egyptian.

The early Hebrews used the zodiac, assigning each of twelve tribes to one of the twelve signs. David Womack's fascinating book *Twelve Signs Twelve Sons*, establishes a possible Israelite origination of the twelve signs. This zodiacal design would have traveled with them into their Babylonian exile. This idea is not without some support. The Biblical King Nebuchadezzar examined the captive Hebrew wise men, declaring them "ten times better" than all of the astrologers of Babylon, our supposed land of origin for astrology ( Daniel, 1:19-20 ).

We know the Egyptians assigned the body parts to the zodiac signs, and invoked the entities in dominion of the signs for assistance with the afflicted corresponding body part. Might the Jewish slaves of Egypt have absorbed some of this Egyptian knowledge, bringing it with them into their Babylonian captivity? Of course, this is mere speculation. Their "host" King Nebuchadnezzar seemed impressed.

The ancient Hebrews were the first to proffer that man was made, both spiritually and physically, in the literal image of his God. Later Jewish thinkers resolved that physical man was the miniature image of God's extended body, the solar system, and more extremely in reverse, that the solar system (God's creation) was actually created in the an image of man!

The Jewish idea of *Adam Kadmon*, the macrocosmic Heavenly Man of the the Solar System and his microcosmic clone, homo sapiens, found its way into Western thinking via the Kabbalistic literature of the late medieval period. Correlations were drawn between the Kabbala's *Tree of Life*, Adam Kadmon and various centers and chakras of the human body.

Physicians of Jewish heritage would have had access to the Kabbalistic idea that our physical body is a solar system in miniature, thus intimately linked with the planets, signs and spatial directions, i.e. the "houses". Medical work was in fact, a traditional trade of Jewish men throughout Europe and the middle East.

Hebrew doctors such as the renowned Maimonides or the brilliant physician-astrologer Nostradamus served the courts of kings and sultans alike throughout the medieval and renaissance eras. Thus the collected astrological and mystic knowledge of the Jews infiltrated European medical practice via the Jewish doctors of the diaspora.

We do know that the scaffold of the system of Medical Astrology as we know it today was in place before Ptolemy outlined medical rules and advice in his *Tetrobiblios*, 140 A.D. It is said that much of his work was copied from far earlier sources at the Library of Alexandria. It is even plausible that a sophisticated lore in this subject was lost when this library was burned, and that what we have today is a mere remnant. It is not impossible to speculate that astrology is far older than assumed and may have ties to an earlier tradition, perhaps Atlantean.

Western physician astrologers continued to innovate through out the centuries, developing new techniques and collecting case studies. They developed this science of astrophysical influence by observing the planetary charts of the ailing, outlining the observed planetary "signatures" for manifold diseases. Medical astrology kept pace with Western medicine's deepening understanding of anatomy. Today's system of planetary correlation to the human body is complex and sophisticated. The flower of this continued development is H. L. Cornell, M.D.'s amazing tome: *The Encyclopedia of Medical Astrology*, 1933.

Planetary correspondences to vitamins and minerals, have been independently assigned by both Eileen Nauman and Robert C. Jansky, introducing the new science of Astro-Nutrition.

Dr. William Davidson's *Davidson's Medical Lectures* is a treasure trove of discourses on novel medical observations and astro-medical discoveries. For instance, he notes Saturn in Libra's role in headaches through an indication of sclerotic kidneys. He gives details on planetary correlation with types of diabetes and how to recognize false diabetes. Such knowledge was heretofore unknown to medical astrologers.

Medical Astrology has long been used to assist in medical diagnosis, and also to time the most effective times for treatment and the safest dates for surgery. Readers seeking direction on the latter will find the enclosed chapter "Selecting Safe Surgery Dates" of inestimable value.

Herbs were assigned to the twelve signs and the seven Ptolemaic planets. The extensive use and designation of herbal-astrological correspondences by the great English herbalist Nicolas Culpeper (1616-1654) are reflected in his words:

"This creation though composed of contraries, is one united body of which man is the epitome, and that he therefore who would understand the mystery of healing, must look as high as the stars".

Medical practitioners prescribed various antidotes designed to balance, absorb or deflect a disharmonious planetary vibration, or to attract one needed. For interest, the author of this book has included a brief section on the Vedic method of gemstone antidotes for planetary conditions.

It is not known why or how the planets and signs influence our bodies. There are many extant theories regarding astral light (Vedic), atmospheric water transference (Buryl Payne, PH.D.), metals resonance (Lily Kolisko, Nick Kollerstrom); vibrational resonance (Judith Hill), amplification of magnetic fields (Percy Seymour).

Physicist Buryl Payne has performed fascinating experiments with astral light and also with magnetism. His theories on how Sunlight influences DNA/RNA or changes the structure of water we drink and breathe are fascinating. For those interested in "How might astrology work?", Payne's works are well worth looking into.

Physicist Lily Kolisko was able to demonstrate, photograph and replicate the metals in salt solution wildly changing under conjunctions of the Moon to the planet that traditionally rules that metal! I think this is key. Nick Kollerstrom outlines Kolisko's astonishing work in his important *The Metal-Planet Relationship* listed in the bibliography.

The efficacy of astral medical science is worth your investment in study time. It has been the experience of the author to see many mysterious cases, after passing unsolved through the offices of multiple doctors be satisfactorily resolved by the medical astrologer. Personally, I've witnessed three lives potentially saved with information obtained from the Planetary Health Chart.

An open minded student will soon see for him/herself how wonderfully accurate and helpful the testimony of planets so often is. After witnessing passes of "heating" Mars over one's ascendant; or observing the planetary transits of a friend's flu bug; or perhaps seeing a baby's congenital respiratory weakness precisely reflected in his birth chart; we know medical astrology works, even if the "how?" remains unknown. Then we come to feel a deep gratitude for all those intrepid and often persecuted practitioners down the centuries who kept this flame alive for us to use, to enhance, and once again, pass on to future generations. This is my reason for writing this book.

# The Planetary Health Chart

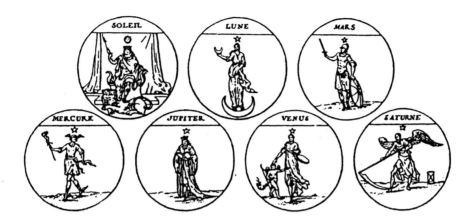

The Planetary Health Chart is calculated using the birth time, date and place of birth. Alternative terms are: "radix", "natal chart", "birth map" and the popular "horoscope". The possessor of the birth map is traditionally referred to as the "native". In medical astrology, this birth map becomes your foremost tool for assessing any "native's" health tendencies, possible timing of disease onset, diagnosis of pathology, suggestion of treatment, selection of herbs and appropriate timing for the administration of medicines or surgery.

How does one begin assessing the Planetary Health Chart for a general description of health tendencies? One of the first things to know is that planetary influence on health is not restricted to the three astrological "houses" of health (1, 6, 8); nor even to the classical evil trio of "malefic" houses (6, 8, 12). Absolutely not. Any afflicted planet, posited in any house of the Planetary Health Chart can demonstrate symptoms aligned to its sign and house position. In some cases, the planet need not even be afflicted! True, a planet in a malefic house is much more likely to demonstrate pathology. Also, a planet ruling a malefic house may become pathological.

There are various approaches to analyzing the Planetary Health Chart and providing a health assessment of that chart. I will define these astrological methods as Nine Key Points of Health Assessment, below.

The following chapters will thoroughly explain these points, and much more. This is a complex study, and as Betty Davis once said of old age, "no place for sissies". Digest each chapter before moving to the next. Understanding the first five "assessments" will enable you to detect areas of potential pathology and guard against it.

**Nine Key Points of Health Assessment Based on the Planetary Health Chart.**

1) The Twelve Signs and Their Designated Rulerships of the Body Parts.

2) Vitality and Metabolism: Sun, Saturn and Mars.

3) The Distribution of the Life Force: The Moon.

4) Temperature: Saturn and Mars: Too Cold/Too Hot.

5) Excess and Deficiency: The Lunar Nodes.

6) Assessment of Bodily Systems: Planets in the Signs and Houses.

7) The Four Elements (i.e. Four Qualities of the Vital Force) in Excess or Deficiency

8) The Three Modes: Rate of Flow of the Vital Force.

9) Current Time Influences: Transits and Progressions.

NOTE TO BEGINNING STUDENTS OF ASTROLOGY

You will need to be conversant with the traditional astrological symbols for the signs and planets and with the general layout of a planetary birth map. This knowledge can be obtained from any solid beginner text on astrology. A list of basic symbols for the signs and planets is provided for you on page 15.

A student needs to possess an *Ephemeris* of planetary motion for the 20th century and also for this present 21st century. You will need to learn to read this ephemeris (not difficult once you know the symbols. However, you may require a one time tutorial from a more advanced student to jump start you). Ephemerides can readily be obtained through any distributor of astrological books. You will need to obtain (or make your own) blank chart forms for the construction of planetary birth charts.

# The Twelve Signs and Their Bodily Correspondences

Before commencing our study of medical astrology it is essential to know the bodily regions governed by each sign. Understanding the energetic influence of every planet through each of the twelve signs is absolutely basic to the rest of our study. This chapter lists the twelve zodiac signs and their physical correspondences.

In such brief listings it is not possible to list all correlations. The aficionado must obtain a copy of Cornell's *Encyclopedia of Medical Astrology*. Later, we will observe the unique energetic action of each planet, and its influence upon each of the twelve signs.

Medical astrology is largely a study of the placements of the birth Sun, Moon and planets in the *signs*, and only secondarily in the *houses* of the Planetary Health Chart.

Before wading into the wonderful world of medical astrology, please obtain a thorough understanding of this present essential chapter, and also "grok" the *Code of Medical Astrology*, in the chapter immediately following.

## WHAT IS A "SIGN" IN CLASSICAL WESTERN ASTROLOGY?

Simply put, a Western astrological *sign* is an Earth season of thirty days. Sure, these Earth seasons bear the names of twelve starry constellations, known as "the zodiac" but are not identical to these star groups, as often misconstrued.

Let us explain this further. There are twelve seasons, or signs, commencing at the Spring equinox. The first day of Spring is an astronomical fact, a precise Sun-Earth relationship. Each day of the Earth year we receive a different angle, amount and quality of Sunlight. This relationship repeats each year exactly as it has for done so for millennia.

Despite the skeptic's complaints that "the constellations have moved backwards since the zodiac was first envisioned!", we know that the Spring equinox is a fixed Sun-Earth relationship, not dependent on the stars above.

Surprise! The *Tropical* zodiac of Western astrologers, does not use a star based sign wheel at all! Certain star groups may once have been used as markers for these twelve earth seasons. Yes, these markers may have moved about twenty some degrees backwards since their inception. This does not alter the most powerful daily event, the Sun-Earth relationship. Each day of the year's wheel, the Earth and Sun align themselves identically as they three thousand years ago. "Zodiac" and "sign" have, over time, come to mean the same thing. However, the word "sign" has many meanings. Yes, it can refer to various slow moving star groups. However, the word "sign", or even "zodiac sign" can also refer, (albeit erroneously) to one of twelve thirty day earth seasons commencing each year at the Spring equinox.

Knowing this, what does it mean to be a "Taurus" in Western astrology? This means you were born between thirty and sixty days after the Spring equinox and sixty to thirty days before the summer solstice!

How about Capricorn, what's that about? Capricorn is the sign beginning on the Winter solstice and extending forward for thirty days. Capricorn babies are positioned between ninety and sixty days before the Spring equinox.

We see that each day of our year the Earth and Sun form a unique slant to each other, providing an actual subtle difference in the quality and quantity of Sunlight received on earth at each specific location.

We cannot live without the Sun, so obviously this dance is outstandingly important. In India, astrology is known as *Jyotish*, the science of light. This seems appropriate. No light on earth is more powerful than the Sun's light and no relationship more light based than the repeating daily shift of earth slant during Earth's orbit of her Sun.

However, Vedic Astrologers of India disregard this equinox/solstice based Tropical wheel in favor an entirely different astrological device - the *Sidereal* zodiac. Sidereal means "star". The Vedic signs are twelve, each of 30° length, and their wheel encompasses 360°, two facts shared with the *Tropical* wheel. The signs of the *Sidereal* zodiac are created by dividing the Earth's ecliptic plane, her orbital path about the Sun. Therefore, the *Sidereal* zodiac is a radically different creation than the *Tropical* zodiac favored in the West. The *Sidereal* zodiac divides space into twelve signs, never referencing the Earth's equinoxes and solstices as structural pivot points of the sign cycle. Again, the *Tropical* zodiac divides the wheel of earth seasons into twelve, and the equinoxes and solstices are the structural pivot points.

The siderealist's twelve divisions of space hold various astrological influences depending on the nearest star constellations. Certainly stars are powerful in their own right, as are star groups. Western astrologers do also use individual stars, in their true positions, for various purposes including health. Bernadette Brady's land mark tome *Brady's Book of Fixed Stars* demonstrates this point gloriously.

Siderealists and skeptics alike delight in proclaiming that Tropical astrologers are foolishly oblivious to the fact that their "zodiac" of stars has moved! Those who make this claim do not realize that Western astrologers are not using the star based zodiac as their foundation for interpretation!

There are some other interesting facts about the Sidereal zodiac. This zodiac is not truly dependent for its existence on star groups, as so is claimed! True, there are various star groups such as "Aries" or "Cancer" near to these twelve equal divisions of ecliptic space known as the Sidereal zodiac. However, no star group, or "zodiac sign" is exactly 30° in length, nor precisely falling within the belt of the ecliptic plane. Some zodiac signs exceed 40°, others are tiny, whereas many are above or below the ecliptic belt. One can only say that these various star groups called "the zodiac" are nearer in proximity to the ecliptic belt than some other constellations. We might assert that the influence of the star groups comes through the Sidereal designations of ecliptic space without in fact precisely occupying those regions.

The Sidereal astrologers of India observe over five possible beginning points for the starting point of their zodiac wheel, or 0° "Aries".

*Note*: Both Tropical and Sidereal astrologers call the start of their sign wheel "0° Aries". To obtain the Sidereal 0° Aries, a number of degrees is first *subtracted* from the Tropical 0° Aries. This subtracted difference is known as the "ayanamsa". There are several ayanamsas to choose from, varying as much as 6° between them.

In India, the correct Sidereal zodiac of preference varies from province to province and an "official" ayanamsa calculation (that of N.C. Lahiri) was sanctioned by the Indian government in recent times. This mess does not invalidate the Sidereal zodiac anymore than disagreements over house systems invalidates that directions (or houses) do have some meaning for planets found therein. Nor does the "which ayanamsa?" conundrum invalidate the real effects of spatial divisions of the ecliptic plane, documented since antiquity by this wonderful and ingenious Sidereal system.

The real problem lies in the fact that many special timing calculations are made from the precise natal degree of the Moon in the Sidereal system. These calculations can vary considerably between two Sidereal zodiacs with starting points six degrees apart! Even one degree can make a big difference in timing events.

Most significantly, the true natal sign or house position of any planet near a cusp may certainly be questioned when using the Sidereal zodiac. Now, a confusion over sign position is a much bigger deal in medical astrology than a confusion over house position! A confident use of the Sidereal zodiac demands a conviction that your preferred ayanamsa is the correct one, and that the alternative Sidereal zodiacs are incorrect.

The Tropical wheel of signs (or earth seasons) holds no such dilemma for the medical astrologer. The Spring equinox is our "0° Aries", the starting point of our wheel. This real astronomical event has not changed since the gears of the Solar System were first set in motion. The practitioner can use this zodiac with confidence that the backward movement of the star groups through the millennia did not alter this yearly Sun-Earth dance, which repeats each day and year down the eons of time.

## THE SIGNS AND THEIR PHYSICAL CORRESPONDENCES

ARIES: Head, skull, cerebrum, motor centers of brain, frontal and lateral lobes, corpus callosum eyes, optic nerves, crystalline lens of eye, eyeballs, upper jaw. Teeth (with Saturn and Taurus). Aries is probably more associated with the teeth of the upper jaw.
(See *Sun in Aries* and *Aries Diseases*, next chapter).

TAURUS: Ears, neck, caratoid arteries, vessels of the neck, salivary glands, lower jaw, sternocleidomastoids, cervical vertebrae, base of skull, cerebellum, chin, taste buds, vocal cords, upper portion of esophagus, tonsils. Hearing (with Gemini). Teeth (with Saturn and Aries. Taurus is associated strongly with the teeth of the lower jaw). Sense of taste (with Mars). The tongue (with Mercury). The nose is under the rule of Scorpio.
(See *Sun in Taurus* and *Taurus diseases* next chapter).

GEMINI: Hands, arms (not elbow), fingers, trachea, bronchial tube, lower esophagus, upper lobes of lungs, scapula, clavicle, pleura (with Cancer), voluntary nerves (with Mercury), speech, hearing (with Taurus).
The capillaries. (See *Sun in Gemini* and *Gemini diseases* next chapter).

CANCER; Stomach (with Moon), mucous membranes in general, breasts and nipples (with Moon), rib cage, elbows, lower lobes of lung, spleen (Carter), gastric mucosa, pleura, some association with meninges of brain and also the fatty protection of eyes, water retention, lower esophagus, upper lobes of liver (Cornell), uterus (see Scorpio), the diaphragm (with

Virgo), temperature regulation of the body.
(See *Sun in Cancer* and *Cancer diseases* next chapter).

LEO: The back in general, the spinal cord, heart, vena cava, aorta. The myelin sheaths.
(See *Sun in Leo* and *Leo diseases* next chapter).

VIRGO: Pancreas, lower lobes of liver, upper intestines, appendix, cecum, ascending colon, abdominal cavity, bile duct, diaphragm, solar plexus, immune system (with Pisces), duodenum (with Pisces - writers vary), spleen (Cornell, but Carter's findings indicate Cancer rules this gland). Some relation to womb with Cancer and Scorpio, the sympathetic nervous system, the solar plexus, the diaphragm (with Cancer).
(See *Sun in Virgo* and *Virgo diseases* next chapter).

LIBRA: Kidneys, lumbar region of back, (Leo is the back in general), acid-alcaline balancing, hormonal balancing, fallopian tubes, reins, distillation and filtration of urine, ovaries (with Venus), veins (with Venus and Aquarius).
(See *Sun in Libra* and *Libra diseases* next chapter).

SCORPIO: Colon, rectum, prostate, anus, bladder, male genitalia, female genitalia, cervix and glandular portion of uterus along with the neck of womb, sweat glands, nose, pelvis, sacrum, coccyx.
(See *Sun in Scorpio* and *Scorpio diseases* next chapter).

SAGITTARIUS: Hips, hip bones, femur, thighs, sciatic nerve, arteries, (with Jupiter), glutteals, some relation to the spinal cord (with Leo). The central nervous system (CNS) is coordinated under Sagittarius, the voluntary peripheral nerves being under the opposite sign Gemini, and the sympathetic peripheral nerves being more under Saturn, according to Cornell. Sagittarius squaring Virgo influences the sympathetic nerves.
(See *Sun in Sagittarius* and *Sagittarius Diseases*, next chapter).

CAPRICORN: Knees, the skin (with Saturn and Venus), sebaceous glands (?), bones, nails and cuticles in general (with Saturn). The teeth are influenced in this sign, although are under the general rulership of Aries (upper teeth), Taurus (lower teeth), and Saturn. The gums are related to the opposite sign Cancer.
(See *Sun in Capricorn* and *Capricorn diseases*, next chapter).

AQUARIUS: Ankles, lower leg, achilles tendon, circulation, veins (with Libra and Venus), oxygenation of blood, the little understood electrical system of the body (with Uranus).
(See *Sun in Aquarius* and *Aquarius diseases*, next chapter).

PISCES: Feet, toes, heel, blood (with Aquarius, Moon and Mars), lymph and lymphatics, duodenum (with Virgo).
(See *Sun in Pisces* and *Pisces diseases*, next chapter).

**Sign Polarity: The Bodily Systems.**

Each sign stands opposite to another sign. This forms a partnership termed a "pole", because these signs stand in polarity. There are six polarities in Medical astrology. Each polarity "governs", i.e. strongly influences certain of the bodily systems.

An emphasis in both signs of a polarity may result in an emphasis witnessed in one or more of the bodily systems described below. Or, a planetary emphasis in one sign of the pole can "reflex" into the opposite sign, producing symptoms truer to the opposite sign! It is better to be medically knowledgeable of your "poles" than of your dominant signs in isolation.

ARIES-LIBRA:   Acid-alkaline balance, glandular balances, adrenals.

TAURUS-SCORPIO: Excretory System - the two poles of the alimentary canal. Food comes in at Taurus and goes out at Scorpio. The Reproductive System.

GEMINI-SAGITTARIUS: The nervous system in general, although the influence is greatest upon the voluntary nerves. The sciatic nerve and central nervous system is largely under the domain of this polarity, also see Virgo. The respiratory system (mostly under Gemini).

CANCER-CAPRICORN: The structural system. Capricorn is the skeletal system and Cancer governs the waters of the body, giving it shape. Nutrient absorption. Food is digested in the stomach (Cancer), and becomes skeletal structure through Capricorn. This pole influences the mucous membranes.

LEO-AQUARIUS: Circulatory System (with Sagittarius which governs the arterial system). The entire pulmonary system is influenced by this polarity.

VIRGO-PISCES: The immune system. The lymphatics. This polarity holds some influence over the sympathetic (involuntary) nervous system. The nervous system in general is under Gemini-Sagittarius.

## The Code of Medical Astrology: Introduction

The Code of Medical Astrology is simple. It has two basic points (points 1 and 2, below). Points 3-10 round out the "Code".
The three basic components of the Code are: *planets, signs and houses.*

**"Planets"** includes the Sun, Moon, Mercury, Venus, Mars, Jupiter, Saturn, Uranus, Neptune, Pluto, Lunar Nodes.

**"Signs"** are the twelve astrological seasons. These are: Aries, Taurus, Gemini, Cancer, Leo, Virgo, Libra, Scorpio, Sagittarius, Capricorn, Aquarius, Pisces. In this text we refer to the Tropical Zodiac.

**"Houses"** are twelve divisions of the horoscope beginning with the ascendant sign which demarcates the 1st house. There are many systems of house division, some based on divisions of space; whereas others, such as Placidus, divide time. The student will prefer his/her habituated house system. The author's favored technique is demonstrated on page 102, #12.

The most important houses for health are the: 1st, 6th, 8th, 12th.

## THE CODE OF MEDICAL ASTROLOGY

1) Planets are the activating energies, describing various types of symptomology and pathology.

2) Signs represent the body parts.

3) Planets in signs suggest <u>what</u> pathological action (the planet) is taking place <u>where</u> in the body (the sign).

4) The signs rule the body in general. However, the planets rule, or sometimes share with the signs rulership over the glands and major organs of the body. This is an important distinction.

5) Planetary action can *reflex* to signs opposing (180°), and squaring (90°). Planetary symptomology can demonstrate itself in the governed body parts of any of these three reflexing signs.

*Note:* In the case of Mars, the Quincunx aspect (150°) is also very strong and the symptomology of Mars can reflect on to the body part governed by the sign Mars quincunxes.

6) Planets are *active* in influence to the signs which are *passive* recipients of planetary energy. However, the sign's quality will alter the planet's nature in four ways: strengthen, weaken, make more positive, make more negative.

*Note:* There are cases where the sign influences the planet rather than the other way around. Keep in mind that this is the exception and not the rule.

*Example*: Saturn in early Pisces might normally indicate a tendency for bone spurs in the heel. Thus, Saturn's calcifying energy impacts the heel, a body part under the rulership of early Pisces, the sign here being recipient of Saturn's energy.

However, the diffusive nature of the sign Pisces can also weaken Saturn, the planetary ruler of the bones - creating osteoporosis or break down of bone tissue, rather the opposite of calcification. In this case (Saturn in Pisces) we might get prolapsed or weak feet.

7) The twelve houses can mimic the twelve signs as parts of the body. Use the sign that corresponds by number to the house. However, the *sign-body correspondences* are primary, and the *house-body correspondences are secondary.* E.g., the sixth sign Virgo corresponds to the sixth house. Both the sign and the house will reflect the health of the upper intestines although the sign Virgo's influence should be observed first. Use old style "a sign for a house" system for counting houses (see Chapter 14).

8) The Planetary Health Chart (Natal Chart read for health purposes) suggests one's health tendencies and natural weaknesses.

Planetary *progressions* indicate when a tendency promised at birth is due, give or take a year.

The current planetary *transits* bring the necessary planetary weather to "hatch" the natal health tendency, and can be timed to within a specific month. Transits work admirably without the collusion of progressions.
It is a great mistake to think you must have a progression to indicate onset. Transits can trigger onset of symptoms all by themselves!

However, if progressions are also involved with transits then the health issue must be given greater weight in one's diagnosis.

9) In most cases the appearance of "promised" health problems can be averted with appropriate prevention before the onset of progressed and transit prompts.

Progressions and transits will be discussed later in Chapters 17 and 19.

10) Not all negative planetary aspects reflect upon the physical level. <u>This is normal.</u> The majority of negative aspects occurring at any given time by transit in anyone's chart, or observed natally, are usually not demonstrating physical symptoms.

Conversely, physical symptoms are almost always accompanied by clear planetary indications, either natally or by transit influence.

## PLANETARY AND SIGN SYMBOLS

| PLANET | | SIGNS | |
|---|---|---|---|
| Sun | ☉ | Aries | ♈ |
| Moon | ☽ | Taurus | ♉ |
| Mercury | ☿ | Gemini | ♊ |
| Venus | ♀ | Cancer | ♋ |
| Mars | ♂ | Leo | ♌ |
| Jupiter | ♃ | Virgo | ♍ |
| Saturn | ♄ | Libra | ♎ |
| Uranus | ♅ | Scorpio | ♏ |
| Neptune | ♆ | Sagittarius | ♐ |
| Pluto | ♇, ♇ | Capricorn | ♑ |
| North Lunar Node | ☊ | Aquarius | ♒ |
| South Lunar Node | ☋ | Pisces | ♓ |
| Pars Fortuna | ⊗ | | |

# The Sun: Life Battery

## The Sun in the Twelve Signs, Diseases of the Signs

The position of the Sun in the Planetary Health Chart (by sign, element, house and aspect) indicates both the *quality* and *quantity* of our natural Vital Force. *See also the Sun's Action and Associations, page 69.*

SUN IN DIGNITY AND DEBILITY
The Sun's natural vital force flows brightly through his signs of *Dignity* (i.e. *rulership* and *exaltation*, below). However, Sol is compromised in his signs of *Debility* (i.e. detriment and fall, below). E.g., the Libran and Aquarius Sun signs (i.e. the Sun's detriment and fall) are seldom as physically vital or as self confident as a strong Leo or Aries Sun sign (Sun's positions of rulership and exaltation).

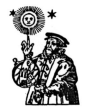

Sun Rules: Leo
Sun Exalted: Aries (best near 19°)
Sun Detriment: Aquarius
Sun Fall: Libra (peaks near 19°)

SUN IN ARIES *March 21st to April 20th*
Element: *Fire*, Mode: *Cardinal*
Ruler: *Mars*

Emphasizes this sign: (See *Aries* bodily regions, previous chapter). Aries is the exaltation of the Sun. The natural vitality is very strong in this sign, moving outward in sudden, sporadic bursts. This is one of the longest - lived signs in two separate studies provided the native does not expire by accident or war. The disease resistance power is very strong. Aries types throw off their toxins. These natives tend to high fevers and fast onset acute conditions. Aries is not prone to the chronic conditions of the more stagnant signs.

Aries diseases and issues: hair lip, wine stains (birth marks), epilepsy, stroke, ringworm, conjunctivitis, acne, gum boils, nervous toothache, headache, fever, cradle cap, baldness, vertigo, accidents, gunshot wounds, convulsions, seizures, aneurism, rash.

SUN IN TAURUS *April 21st to May 20th*
Element: *Earth;* Mode: *Fixed*
Ruler: *Venus*

Emphasizes this sign. (See *Taurus* bodily regions, previous chapter). This sign steadies and enhances vitality. Taurus is the longest lived of all the signs in two separate research studies. This sign provides its natives with huge magnetic energy. The life force burns slowly in this birth season. The Taurus native is very strong, healthy, tough, and has fine resistance. However, they are prone to chronic conditions later in life due to a tendency to overeating of rich and sweet foods. Taurean types tend to hold toxins within the body.

Taurus diseases and issues: Overweight, goiter, hypo thyroid, quinsy, gout, toxemia from gormandizing, throat colds, deafness, ear infections, excess mucous in ear-nose-throat, gorging, congested colon, tonsillitis, vocal chord afflictions, dental issues, problems of the esophagus.

SUN IN GEMINI *May 21st to June 20th*
Element: *Air;* Mode: *Mutable*
Ruler: *Mercury*

Emphasizes this sign. (See *Gemini* bodily regions, previous chapter). Geminian vital force is a bit scattered, reminiscent of a breeze blowing about in several directions.

Natives of this playful birth season will be quite healthy if they eat correctly, and get enough rest. However, they seldom do either. The nervous system is overactive in this sign and needs to be nourished.

The quality of the vital force in Gemini depends on how strained and depleted the natives of this sign allow themselves to become. Gemini natives need to be watched closely when ill, as they are prone to lingering ailments which go unchecked until too late, such as tuberculosis. The lungs need extra attention.

Gemini issues and diseases: nervous diseases, speech impediments, learning disorders, carpal tunnel syndrome, neurological problems and accidents to the shoulders, arms and hands, pneumonia, bronchitis, asthma, under eating, junk food addictions, media and computer addiction, neurological burn-out, mental illness.

SUN IN CANCER *June 21st to July 22nd*
Element: *Water;* Mode: *Cardinal*
Ruler: *Moon*

Emphasizes this sign. (See *Cancer* bodily regions previous chapter). The life force is notably weak in this sign, especially in children. The Cancer native is wise to guard his life force like gold. Most Cancers accomplish this by taking frequent retreats from people and life. Naps are needed! Too much sunshine, exercise or physical work is straining to the natives of Cancer. These people seem to perform best by Moonlight. The lungs, stomach, glandular and female system need tonification.

Cancer diseases and issues: Eating disorders, food neurosis, overweight, underweight, anorexia, edema, swollen breasts, brain chemistry imbalance, depression, sensitive teeth or gums, sun intolerance, weak stomach, weak lungs, paranoia, lack of exercise, fatigue, allergies.

SUN IN LEO *July 23rd to August 22nd*
Element: *Fire;* Mode; *Fixed*
Ruler: *Sun*

Emphasizes this sign: (See *Leo* bodily regions, previous chapter). This is the Sun's home sign, giving excellent vitality. Leos have tremendous life force which they tend to misspend in the wild pleasure sprees of youth. A front runner is not always at the finish line, so be wise! Leos need to drink lots of pure water. More than any other, Leo is prone to dehydration.

Leo diseases and issues: Heart disease, hypertension, syncopes, eye diseases, convulsions, excessive meat eating, alcoholism, backache, scoliosis, diseases of the spinal cord nerve sheaths, dehydration, heatstroke, stroke.

SUN IN VIRGO *August 23rd to September 22nd*
Element: *Earth;* Mode: *Mutable*
Ruler: *Mercury*

Emphasizes this sign: (See *Virgo* bodily regions, previous chapter). This is a wiry and yet hardy sign with great stamina. The writer has always thought that the dutiful, burden bearing donkey was a better symbol than a virgin holding a sprig of grain!

Nevertheless, the Virgo vital force requires careful maintenance and great attention to the diet and digestive organs. This is generally not a problem because most Virgo natives are interested, (if not obsessed) with their health and nutrition. The energy movement of the chi force is quick, highly strung and yet simultaneously strong and enduring. This wiry, dainty and coordinated sign makes excellent gymnasts and yogis.

Virgo diseases and issues: diverticulitis, diabetes, hepatitis, colitis, worms, dysentery, hernia, insomnia, appendicitis, anxiousness, premature gray.

SUN IN LIBRA *September 23rd to October 22nd*
Element: *Air;* Mode: *Cardinal*
Ruler: *Venus*
Emphasizes this sign. (See *Libra* bodily regions, previous chapter).
The vitality of Libra is excellent and the natives are rarely sick. Many Librans demonstrate a curious ability of being able to live off sugar and junk food for years, appearing none the worse for it. Libra gives a relaxed, easy going chi force and muscular strength independent of exercise. The love of sugar and utter disregard of the laws of health may eventually undo them, as the kidneys and alkaline balance of the blood are sensitive in this sign. Libra would perhaps be the healthiest sign of all, if only its natives took an interest in health matters!

Libra diseases and issues: Sugar addiction, alcoholism, acne, kidney disease, glandular imbalance, dizziness, acid-alkaline imbalance, adrenal issues, lumbago, venereal disease, ovarian problems.

SUN IN SCORPIO *October 23rd to November 22nd*
Element: *Water;* Mode: *Fixed*
Planet Ruler: *Mars* (traditional), and *Pluto* (recently assigned)
Emphasizes this sign. (See *Scorpio* bodily regions, previous chapter). The Chi force is very powerful in this sign and Scorpio's children can overcome even the most serious and life threatening of illnesses. Scorpio has more than one life and will always rise again!

This sign throws off toxins. Intense body odor, acne, poisoned blood, surliness and diarrhea are possible outcomes of this tendency. Scorpios need assistance in this "detoxing" process with alterative herbs, sweat baths, etc. There is some tendency in this birth season toward long term and chronic ailments that must be battled, usually successfully. This is the internally strongest, and often externally toughest of all signs.

*continued next page*

<u>Scorpio diseases and issues</u>: Venereal disease, mennoraghia, prostitis, hemorrhoids, bladder infection, parasites, colitis, Crone's disease, excessive sweating, obsessions, uterine issues, candida, piles, fistulas, hernias, diarrhea, glandular excesses, STDs, uterine fibroids.

SUN IN SAGITTARIUS *November 23rd through December 21st*
  <u>Element: *Fire;* Mode: *Mutable*</u>
<u>Ruler: *Jupiter*</u>

Emphasizes this sign. (See *Sagittarius* bodily regions, previous chapter). The vital force is vigorously outward moving. There is much vital energy in the both the muscular and nervous systems, creating a rather restless kinetic individual in many cases. These people are spark plugs.

Always on the go, natives of this sign burn the candle at both ends and suffer for it in their later years. Like their mascot the horse, they require sufficient leg exercise and fresh air. This is a healthy sign if the blood pressure is regulated and bodily structure, (particularly of the spine, hips and legs) is maintained.

<u>Sagittarius diseases and issues:</u> Injuries from: sports, horse riding, hunting and driving. Spinal issues, sciatica, diseases of spinal cord or central nervous system, hysteria, grandiosity, ADHD, heated blood, high blood pressure, fevers, fits, gunshot wounds, fire, hip problems, structural misalignments of spine and hip, insomnia, eye problems, disordered and depleted system from too much activity or travel, mental derangement.

SUN IN CAPRICORN *December 22nd to January 19th*
  <u>Element: *Earth;* Mode: *Cardinal*</u>
<u>Ruler: *Saturn*</u>

Emphasizes this sign. (See *Capricorn* bodily regions, previous chapter).

The vitality of Capricornians is fragile in childhood and strong in age. The candle of Capricornian vital force is faint at first and slow burning. However, the flame strengthens and brightens as years goes by!

Colicky and croupy Capricornian infants may require extra attention to their diet, and skin. The Capricornian must be diligent and make sure that even common colds do not work into more serious problems. Capricornians are wise to adopt a nutritional program tailored to their special requirements and also, to absolutely maintain the moisture of the mucous lining of the entire intestinal tract and the skin. Beware of under eating and malnourishment. Frequent small meals seem best, as goats do.

Above all signs, Capricorn is sensitive to oils: the right kind are very needed and the wrong kind will do great damage to natives of this birth season. The liver and gall bladder seem sluggish in this sign, and may need frequent cleansing. Toxic build up should never be allowed in Capricorns, who are prone to rheumatic and skin disorders related to toxic conditions and/or a lack of natural moisture and protective skin oils.

Calcium balance is essential for those born in this sign. There the nails, cuticles and teeth appear more susceptible than average to complaints. In adulthood, this sign is surprisingly strong and tough. Muscular strength is often outstanding.

In their advanced years, the leaner type Capricorn demonstrates fantastic endurance and can live on groats! The older Capricorn, if not arthritic, can be observed happily pottering around in the garden or doing carpentry projects when their stronger brethren of other signs are long out to pasture.

Capricorn diseases and issues: Rheumatism, arthritis, knee problems, skin disease, dryness of mucous membrane, infertility, cuticle complaints, warts, moles, brittle nails, nail fungus, freckles, leprosy, keloids, mineral and vitamin deficiency, trick knee, fractures, bad teeth and gums, falling, chronic malnutrition, anorexia, constipation, uterine complaints.

SUN IN AQUARIUS *January 20th to February 19th*
Element: *Air;* Mode: *Fixed*
 *Ruler*: *Saturn* (traditional), and *Uranus* (modern assignment)

Emphasizes this sign, (See *Aquarius* bodily regions, previous chapter). The Sun "falls" in this sign and thus we can expect a weaker vital force. Aquarians seem uniquely prone to light deficiency, fatigue, depression and anemia. However, many are excellent athletes anyway.

The vital force in this sign is electrical and erratic - appearing in spasmodic spurts, or power surges of energy followed by periods of low force on all levels. Planets in Fire signs will counterbalance these tendencies.

Natives of this sign are influenced by electromagnetic fields more than any other birth month, and are wise to investigate the strength of adverse electromagnetic fields before selecting living environments and careers. *continued next page*

Aquarian vital force can be easily depleted through excessive involvement in computers and other electromagnetically toxic devices, or exposure to fluorescent lighting. The upper body should be strengthened. Davidson cites that no sign is more responsive to barometric changes than is Aquarius.

The Aquarian native needs to build a strong heart muscle. Generally speaking, Aquarians are "healthy" and rarely sick with normal, everyday ailments; instead, their problems are often puzzling and difficult to diagnose. Salt is important for natives of this sign (salt conducts electricity). The Aquarian nervous system needs restful, soothing influences.

Aquarius diseases and issues: Anemia, nervous sensitivity, muscle spasms, blood poisoning, insufficient blood, ankle swelling, varicose veins, weak heart, rheumatism, cold extremities, weird "undiagnosable" ailments, fatigue, spasmodic diseases, low blood pressure, computer addiction, mental extremes.

SUN IN PISCES: *Feb. 19th to March 21st.* Element: *Water;* Mode: *Mutable* Ruler: *Jupiter* (traditional), and *Neptune* (modern assignment)

Emphasizes this sign. (See *Pisces* bodily regions, previous chapter). The vital force is notably diffused in this sign. The Piscean is psychically delicate and may experience weakness on several levels. Often they are barely here, with one foot in the astral world. Healthy Pisceans are flexible, easy going, cheerful and extremely multifaceted. Piscean chi benefits from warmth, stimulation and useful projects.

The Piscean Sun or Moon native requires more sleep than natives of other signs. Most Pisceans take plenty of retreat time to diffuse their consciousness away from worldly stress and house work.

As a rule, a Pisces shows poor recuperative ability and needs all the help he/she can get. Special care must be taken to not allow small issues to take hold. Pisceans must never drink or take drugs because unnatural substances impact them more profoundly than most signs, and may lead to death. The immune system is weak and Pisceans need to protect themselves with antiviral and antibacterial herbs. Nutritives are essential. Pisceans respond well to gentle, diffusive and holistic treatments that address the entire system (homeopathy, herbology, nutritives, foot reflexology).

It is completely natural and healthful for natives of this sign to eschew hard labor and sleep late. Pisceans need plenty of decompression time. *continued next page*

<u>Pisces diseases and issues:</u> Sleepiness, painful feet, shoe sensitivities, (e.g. dislike of enclosed shoes, collecting shoes, etc.), weakness, lung sensitivity, edema, obesity, glandular issues affecting height and size, lymphatic swelling, weak immunity, overeating, foot problems, narcolepsy, depression, excessive sex drive, boils, itch and eruptions from corrupted blood, mucous discharges.

## THE DEGREES: Fine Tuning the Signs

Each Sign is divided into thirty days, or degrees. Each degree relates to a body part or specific disease. Take the circle of twelve signs (360 degrees) and "unsnip" the circle as if it were a string and hang it vertically as in a line. The top of the string becomes, 0° Aries, and rules the very top of the head. The last degree, the end of the string, is 360° - the last degree of the last sign, Pisces. This degree governs the tips of the toes. All other degrees fall in between!

Take Aries for example, which governs the skull through the upper jaw, inclusive of the eyes. The first third (10°) of Aries governs the first third of this region, the second third the middle portion, and the last decanate, or third of Aries rules the lower portion of Aries' region, inclusive of the upper portion of the jaw bone.

Let us now examine the last sign Pisces, because it is easy. Pisces rules "the feet". We can fine tune this more precisely. The first ten degrees, or one third of Pisces influences the heel bones. The second decanate of Pisces governs the mid foot. The last ten degrees of this sign governs the toes. Similarly, the first third of Scorpio governs the upper portion of the Scorpio region: the uterus and bladder, while the last third of Scorpio governs the anus.

The best of the various degree systems was established by Elsbeth and Reinhold Ebertin in their *Anatomische Entsprechungen Der Tierkreisgrade*. I have located two English language reproductions of this material (below). It would be very, very worth your time to obtain a copy of this degree system.

A brief list of degrees of observed correspondence to disease conditions below. My four sources are: Donna Walter Henson (her book *Degrees of the Zodiac* is a must!), C.E.O. Carter, Nicholas Devore, the Ebertins, plus my case files. These authors are listed in the bibliography.

This list of Disease Degrees is woefully incomplete! Obviously someone's pet research diseases were rheumatism, Bright's disease, eyesight, neuritis, and appendicitis. Little attention is paid to the remaining gamut of mankind's travails. To hinder matters further, no source with the exceptions of Carter and Henson, mention their own sources; and if they do, fail to describe their source's methods for obtaining these degree associations! For all we know, some of these degrees could have arisen from the "case files" of one example from some "researching" astrologer of antiquity. I can vouch only for the veracity of the "appendicitis degrees" near 16-19° Virgo and Scorpio because my own handful of case studies make me a believer.

Despite all these problems with traditional degree lists, we do have a start! Future research by intrepid degree freaks will reveal more about degree sensitivities.

To obtain "Anatomical Correspondences to Zodiacal Degrees":
*A Handbook of Medical Astrology* by Jane Ridder-Patrick.
ISBN: 0 14 01.9214 X

"The NCGR Journal", Winter 85-86, Volume 4, no. 2 (Medical Edition), translated by Mary L. Vohryzek.
Contact: The National Council for Geocosmic Research

DISEASE DEGREES
*Note: These degrees are read from the listed degree. Example: 9° includes the precise area between 9-10°.*

ARIES: 3-4°: goiter; 9-12°: fevers; 6-7°: jaundice; 13-14°: rheumatic fever, rheumatism; hemorrhage, 15-16°: stroke; 20-21°: abscesses; 25-26°: tuberculosis, digestive troubles; 26-27°: blindness; weak eyes; 28-29°: bronchitis.

TAURUS; 0-6°: drowning; 8-9°: alcoholism; 9-13°: neurasthenia; 17-18°: appendicitis;19-23°: alcoholism; 19-20°: goiter; 22-23°: defective sight, rheumatism; 24-25°: fractures, broken bones, alcoholism; 27-28°: alcoholism.

GEMINI: 3-4°: pulmonary inflammation; 9-10°: typhoid fever; 12-13° : rheumatic fever; 14-15°: muteness or impaired organs of speech;15-16° : asthma, lung trouble, pneumonia; 16°: AIDS (Millard); 16-19°: Bright's disease, sleep and trance; 17-18°: asthma; 18-23°: defective sight, eye troubles; 21-22°: appendicitis; 24-26°: neurasthenia; 27-28°: tuberculosis; 29-30°: angina pectoris, gastric ulcer; 24-25°: duodenal ulcer; 27-28°: digestive troubles, tuberculosis, 28-30°: depression.

CANCER: 0-1°: drowning, eyesight; 5-6°: sleep and trance; 10-12°: alcoholism; 12-13°: associated with dog bites; 14-15°: blindness or defective sight; 17-19°: chemicals, poisons and gas; 22-23°: weak or impaired vision; 24-25°: danger through water, gas, poisons, dog bites; 27-28°: digestive troubles; 27-30°: depression, mental and emotional difficulties and instability; 28-29°: the spleen; 29-30°: bronchitis.

LEO: 7-8°: anemia, fevers; 8-9°: burns; 9-10°: bladder afflictions, alcoholism; 22-23°: appendicitis; 23-24°: appendicitis, rheumatism; 25-28°: poisoning, drowning, asphyxiation; 26-27°: goiter; 28-29°: neuritis.

VIRGO: 4-5°: asthma; 9-10°: rheumatic fever; 14-15°: emphasis on feet; 16-18°: appendicitis; diabetes; 22-23°: appendicitis; 23-24°: defective vision; 24-25°: cancer, gout, arthritis; 25-26°: gout, cancer, neurasthenia; 27-28°: Bright's disease, excema, tuberculosis, diabetes; 28-29°: drowning, consumption.

LIBRA: 3-4°: abscesses; 4-5°: goiter; 6-7°: goiter; 7-11°: jaundice of the kidney and renal pelvis; 15-16°: excema, stroke; 18-19°: Bright's disease; 26-27°: tuberculosis; 27-28°: tuberculosis; 28-29°: bladder trouble; 29-30°: bronchitis.

SCORPIO: 0-6°: drowning; 10-11°: neurasthenia; 11-12°: Bright's disease; 14-15°: danger of poison; 16-17°: abscesses; 18-19°: appendix; 20-22°: danger of poison; 23-24°: rheumatism; 24-25°: alcoholism; 25-26°: alcoholism, adenoids, muteness, tonsils, fractures, broken bones; 27-28°: memory, poisons; 28-29°: consumption, poisons, stings, depression; 29-30°: blindness, impaired vision, depression, stings, poisons.

SAGITTARIUS: 2-3°: susceptible to contagious diseases; 3-4°: appendicitis; 6-7°: pneumonia; 10-11°: typhoid; 16-17°: sciatic nerve; AIDS (Millard); 19-20°: lungs emphasized or sensitive to smoke; 21-22°: speech impediments; 22-23°: appendicitis; 25-26°: neurasthenia, gout, blindness, impaired sight; 28-29°: impaired eyesight, tuberculosis.

CAPRICORN: 0-3°: blindness; 4-5°: sleep and trance; 8-9°: impaired vision; 11-12°: alcoholism; 14-15°: impaired vision; 17-18°: diabetes; 27-29°: severe depression; 29-30°: bronchitis.

AQUARIUS: 0-1°: danger from reptiles; 1-2°: fatty degeneration; 2-3°: obesity; 8-9°: anemia; 12-13°: bites from venomous creatures; 13-14°: rheumatism; rheumatic fever; 17-19°: Bright's disease; 20-26°: alcoholism; 22-23°: appendicitis; 23-24°: poisoning, rheumatism; 25-26°: alcoholism; 26-27°: neurasthenia; poisoning; 27-28°: goiter; poisoning; 29-30°: neuritis.

PISCES: 3-4°: appendicitis; 4-5°: asthma; 9-10°: rheumatic fever; 11-12°: Bright's disease; 19-20°: digestive ailments or excessive eating; 21-22°: typhoid fever; 22-23°: appendicitis, fevers; 23-24°: fevers; 25-26°: gout, neurasthenia, cancer; 27-28°: eczema, Bright's disease, acute nephritis; 28-29°: diabetes, low blood sugar, bleeding (difficulty clotting), depression; 29-30°: bleeding (difficulty clotting), depression, drowning.

# Metabolism: Sun, Mars and Saturn

Davidson asserts that a natal *aspect* (i.e. geometric relationship) between *Sun and Mars* speeds up the metabolism. A square aspect (90°) between the Sun and Mars is excessive. A Sun-Mars conjunction could have a similar effect. Sun-Mars individuals lose heat quickly, and are frequently hungry. They need to eat frequent, small meals and keep warm.

Conversely, a *Sun-Saturn* aspect slows the metabolism, holds in heat and burns fuel slowly. The appetite is not as robust as with the Sun-Mars aspect.

The conjunction, square or opposition (180°) between Sun and Saturn excessively slows the metabolism, unless balanced. A Sun in Aries or similar could offset this.

It is never clear which way the metabolism swings should you be born with both above conditions simultaneously! Should Saturn and Mars both aspect your Sun, then you have several alternate ways of deciding if the metabolism swings faster or slower.

First, tally the number of planets (through Saturn) in the fast - metabolizing "masculine" signs of the Fire and Air elements (see - below). Compare these with the total number of planets (through Saturn) in the slow metabolizing "feminine" Earth and Water signs. Fire is the fastest element and Earth is the slowest.

Next, note if your ascendant sign is in a Fire or Air sign (fast) or, Earth or Water (slow).

Finally, observe the number of planets (through Saturn) in certain slow - metabolizing Saturn and Venus ruled Signs in this order of slowness: (Capricorn, Taurus, Aquarius). Compare this result with the number of planets (through Saturn) in the fast metabolizing Mars and Sun ruled signs, in this order of speed: (Aries, Leo, Scorpio).

*Result:* A majority of planets in the masculine signs and/or the Mars and Sun ruled signs incline toward a faster metabolism. Conversely, more planets in the feminine and/or Saturn and Venusian signs (except Libra), testifies to a slower metabolism.

## CALORIES AND MARS

The planet Mars governs the speed at which we burn calories. Mars acts slowest in Earth signs, contributing to weight gain. An earthy Mars requires less fuel and burns it slowly compared with a fast Fire Mars. The next slowest element for Mars is Water. Air signs are moderately fast positions.

## THE ELEMENTS AND THE SPEED OF THE METABOLISM

**FIRE SIGNS**: (masculine, very fast) Aries, Leo, Sagittarius.

**AIR SIGNS**: (masculine, moderately fast) Gemini, Libra.
*Note:* Aquarius being a Saturn ruled Air sign may not always behave as do brother masculine signs because Saturn is slow moving and cold. This Saturnian effect seems to outlet itself upon the circulation of Aquarian people whom are famous for their cold hands and feet.

**EARTH SIGNS**: (feminine, very slow) Taurus, Virgo, Capricorn.

**WATER SIGNS**: (feminine, moderately slow) Cancer, Scorpio, Pisces.
*Note*: Scorpio, being a Mars ruled Water sign possesses the fastest metabolism of the Water trio and therefore may not behave as sluggishly as do sister feminine signs.

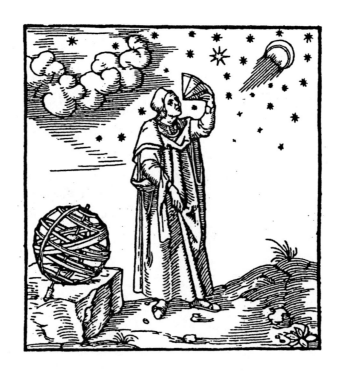

# The Moon: Distributor of the Life Force

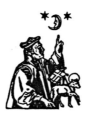

The Moon translates and distributes the light of the Sun. William Davidson M.D. in *Davidson's Medical Lectures,* likens the Sun to our natural voltage of energy and the Moon to our amperage, or rate of flow.

"...I ascribe the the voltage or power of the general metabolism to the Sun, its sign, and aspects, and that I explained that the Moon largely influenced health because it ruled the amperage, or rate of flow - the rhythm, of the inflowing vitality. But there is a third factor which needs consideration, and that is the ascendant sign. In an ordinary electric circuit you have the flow of the current (voltage) the you have the rate of flow (even or uneven) amperage, but there is also the resistance of the wire. Now the physical body, indicated by the ascendant sign, shows the kind of conductivity, or resistance, which the physical body offers. It will thus readily be seen why a Capricorn ascendant (Saturn slowed up) offers more resistance, than in the average hence it is that these youngsters are rarely robust in infancy but mysteriously grow more vigorous as they grow older."

The waters of the Earth are largely the dominion of the Moon. She pulls at the oceans and produces the waves and the tides. Understanding the importance of our birth chart's Moon sign is easy by remembering that our bodies are over 80% water! The Moon's motion creates the vast ocean tides. How can she not then, pull upon our brains, blood vessels, glands and cells? Is it not then evident why above all else, the Moon rules responsiveness and everyday adjustment and change to all manner of stimuli? Our method of self defense is also indicated by our Moon's sign.

Our Moon's birth sign will foretell what part of our body is particularly *sensitive* to light, temperature, and fluidic changes. This sign describes how successfully we adapt to change and also our level of moisture. The emotional tone is indicated. The Moon governs the menses, stomach, mammary glands, meninges ofthe brain, left eye for males (reverse for females) and the lungs (with Gemini and Cancer). Our very word month means a "moonth".

*See Also the Moon's Actions and Associations, page 70:*

MOON IN DIGNITY AND DEBILITY

The Moon's moisturizing and adaptability functions are weakest when in her sign of detriment, Capricorn and suffers emotional troubles in her sign of fall, Scorpio. She is more productive of moisture and fertility in her signs of *dignity i.e.* (rulership and exaltation), but also more inclined to produce growths. She is happiest in Taurus (exaltation).

Moon Rules: Cancer
Moon Exalted: Taurus (best at 4°)
Moon Detriment: Capricorn
Moon Fall: Scorpio (4° is the strongest Fall).
*Note*: The natural energy of Luna is considerably altered in dry, hot Aries.

MOON IN ARIES: The vital force distributes itself in bright, enthusiastic yet short-lived bursts. Responsiveness is immediate and feisty. The Moon Sign speeds up the vital force as shown by the Sun sign.

Dryness of hair, skin and mucous membrane, swelling of brain, light sensitive vision, baldness, cradle cap, itch, headache, insomnia, muscular activity in sleep, disturbed posterior pituitary, ammenorrhia, infertility, miscarriage, temper fits.

MOON IN TAURUS: The vital force distributes itself in a calm and steady manner, but may require stimulation to prevent stagnation .

Sweet tooth, mucous congestion in ears, nose and throat, double chin, soft teeth, overeating, thyroid sensitivity, eye disorders near 29° Taurus, slow metabolism, sugar addiction, edema, obesity, excessive breast tissue, food addictions.

MOON IN GEMINI: The vital life force distributes itself in an irregular and jumpy manner, like changeable breezes. The flow is largely to the nervous system, mind, verbal centers and hands.

Nervousness, mental instability, difficulty being treated with chemical drugs, sensitive or weak shoulders, delicate nerves, arm and finger nerves, weak lung, edema of lungs, pneumonia, asthma, nervous stomach. Gemini Moon people require nerve tonics and if possible, and should avoid chemical drugs.

MOON IN CANCER: The vital force moves inward, into the emotions, womb and stomach. The flow of force appears highly reactive and receptive to incoming influences. The emotional life, brain chemistry, hormones and general health may change abruptly in response to external conditions. The responsiveness is so great in this sign that the native may appear fearful or defensive. These natives need to feel safe and protected.

Painful breasts, skin sensitivity to sun, emotions upset stomach, dropsy, edema, uterine fibroid, breast cysts, nearsightedness, allergies, sensitive eyes, demonstrates a high sensitivity to the changing conditions of: altitude, weather, seasonal and Moon phase. The health is a little sensitive with this Moon position. It is okay to baby yourself.

MOON IN LEO: The vital force distributes itself with concentrated power, warmth and joy. There can be an excess build up of heat within the system. The native may disguise their pains and/or refuse medical help.

Weak back, circulatory disorders, vision issues, backache, dehydration, infertility.

MOON IN VIRGO: The vital force distributes itself quickly yet steadily and in a somewhat finicky manner. Never overload the digestive tract.

Sensitive digestion, hypochondria, dysentery, leaky gut syndrome, under active liver and/or digestive enzymes, blood sugar issues, appendicitis (16-23°), allergies, overwork. Emotions disturb the digestive tract.

MOON IN LIBRA: The vital force "rests" in this sign, creating a pleasant and easygoing effect in these natives. Balances of mind, perception or hormones may be too easily upset in response to outside stimulation.

Abcesses, kidney troubles, glandular imbalance, dizziness, uremia, headaches (reflex from Aries). Observe temperance in all things!

MOON IN SCORPIO: The vital force distributes itself in a concentrated and highly intense manner, largely flowing into the emotional and sexual systems, though not uncommonly transformed towards spiritual efforts.

Uterine fibroid, prostrate congestion, candida, yeast infections, vaginitis, leaky gut syndrome, bladder complaints, incontinence, hydrocele, overactive colon, runny nose, excessive sweating, emotional obsessions, swollen testicles, sensitive genitals, jock itch, hemorrhoids.

*continued next page*

*Scorpio continued*

Persons with a Scorpio Moon position need to carefully maintain their acid/alkaline balance and staunchly minimize "soupy" and bacterial inviting conditions of the genito-urinary tract and colon.

MOON IN SAGITTARIUS: The vital force distributes itself outwardly, sometimes scattering, often into mental flights of fancy, interests or vision. The Moon in this sign acts as a stepping up transformer to the life force. The effect is a restless and positive in quality. If the Sun is weak, the Sagittarian Moon native may throw out more vital force than they have in the bank! These natives flee under restraint or pressure.

Restlessness, insomnia, sciatic sensitivity, cysts in hip or thigh region, paralysis, mental health problems (flights, fantasy, visions, voices), sexual compulsions (satyriasis, infidelity).

MOON IN CAPRICORN: The vital force may become obstructed in this sign and too cold. Persons with this Moon position need to be extra attentive to their physical and emotional health. The vital force expends itself conservatively, giving excellent stamina and endurance.

Uterine complaints (primary sign for this), bleeding gums, weak teeth, osteoporosis, insufficient milk, infertility, fibroids, skin sensitivity to sun, excema, skin disease, dry mucous membrane, weak stomach, poor absorption of nutrients, deficiency in synovial fluid, rheumatism. Obsessive weeping, craving for baths and water. Hysterectomy is a common tendency for this Moon position.

MOON IN AQUARIUS: The vital force distributes itself erratically in power surges and power outages. The life force flows readily into the mental body, enlivening the aspirations and imagination.

Nervous strain, depression, edema of ankles, cold extremities, low blood pressure, dropsy, sensitivity of achilles and ankles, erratic swings of energy, mood and libido, varicose veins, syncope, anemia, fatigue, electromagnetic poisoning, muscle spasms, stiffness, gender identity disorder, puzzling electrical disturbances of nervous system and muscles. These natives are sensitive to changes in barometric pressure.

Individuals with this Moon position need to rest their nerves and frequently remove themselves from all electromagnetic and social influences. Crowds, sudden noise and chaos tends to deplete their vital force.

MOON IN PISCES: The vital force is distributed in a sleepy, meandering, and vague manner. This Moon sign appears to diffuse the vital force of the Sun's sign and slow it down. Stimulants and exercise may be required to offset this tendency.

These natives tend to procrastinate, and when pressured, prefer to escape reality. They are accepting of others and sweet natured.

Swollen feet, boils, swollen lymph glands, weak lungs, immune susceptibility, depression, drug addictions, fatigue, edema, obesity, psychic problems, nymphomania, mennoraghia. The life force moves drowsily through this sign.

The psychic and sexual life accumulate much of the energy from the Sun when the Moon is found in Pisces.

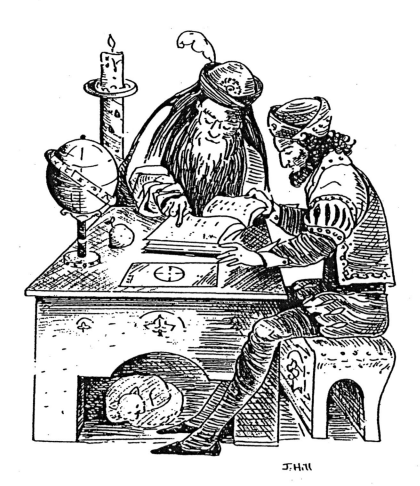

J. Hill

# Saturn and Mars: The Malefics

Saturn and Mars are the *malefics,* i.e. bad guys of classical western astrology. One of the best methods for Health Assessment is the careful observation Saturn and Mars for their effects through astralic temperature extremes upon the human body. In this chapter we will describe HOW to look at cold Saturn first, then hot Mars. Each planet will be followed by a tour through the diseases potentially related to their positions through the twelve signs.

### SATURN - WHERE ILL HEALTH BEGINS

No rule in medical astrology is absolute. That being said, we can safely state that most disease, most of the time, begins with the astrological indications of Saturn's placement in the natal chart. Mars and the South Node are also contenders for this dubious honor. However, Saturn is foremost! Never put this out of your mind.

The human body does not do well with too much cold (Saturn); or too much heat (Mars). We can also think of Saturn as a dark blue color ray, and Mars as red. The human body does not do well under prolonged exposure to light of either color! Remember this essential paragraph and you will understand why these two planets may so easily turn malefic.

Saturn governs the chronic conditions (cold, blue) and Mars is lord of the acute (hot, red).

### HOW TO ASSESS SATURN FOR POTENTIAL HEALTH PATHOLOGY.
### SATURN IN DIGNITY AND DEBILITY

Study Saturn, his sign, condition of strength and house. Write down the sign he is in. Counting the ascendant sign itself as "1", now count the number of signs counter clockwise that Saturn is from the Ascendant. This is his house position in the Planetary Health Chart - write it down. You should now have the sign and house position of Saturn. Now you must decide if Saturn is strong, weak or afflicted. He is strongest in his natural traits when posited in *rulership* or *exaltation*, whereas his native qualities are weakest in *fall* or *detriment*. Saturn in Leo appears an exception.

Saturn Rules: Capricorn and Aquarius. (enhances natural quality)
Saturn Exalted: Libra. (enhances natural quality. Best at 21º)
Saturn in Detriment: Cancer and Leo (alters natural quality)
Saturn in Fall: Aries. (alters natural quality. Peaks at 21º)

*Note:* Does Saturn receives a number of squares, quincunxes or oppositions? If so, consider Saturn a major causative precursor to a disease condition.

SATURN RULES: The bones and skeletal structure in general; the teeth (with Taurus); the skin (with Venus); the nails, cuticles, calcium, minerals (in general), the ear. According to Cornell, he governs the peripheral sympathetic nerves. It is said that Saturn rules the right ear and Mars the left ear. However, the general rulership of the ears is under Taurus, and the sense of hearing under Mercury.

PHYSICAL EFFECTS OF SATURN: Cold, constricts, limits circulation, restricts, undernourishes, paves the way for toxic buildup and stiffness. Saturn can indicate structural anomalies, under function or undersize of any body part indicated. *See Also Saturn's Associations, page 71.*

   Positively: Saturn rules our structure and bones. He can indicate great strength and endurance in the body part indicated.

   *Note:* People with Saturn in the first two houses, (especially in Leo, Taurus or Scorpio) are often extremely strong. Saturn also represents dark blue light, a neurologically strengthening color that should not be used too long on the human body.

*SPECIAL CONDITIONS OF SATURN: IMPORTANT!*

   If you are born at *night*, (with the Sun under the horizon); while Saturn is *simultaneously* posited under the horizon, (where his energy is more concealed); *and* also your Saturn is in a female sign (listed below); then your Saturn is *extremely cold* in temperature, and you must keep an eye on him for sure! If any one of the three above conditions exists, i.e. night birth, Saturn under the horizon, or Saturn in a feminine sign, then your Saturn is colder and/or more sluggish than if these same conditions did not hold. (The feminine signs are: Taurus, Cancer, Virgo, Scorpio, Capricorn, Pisces).

   However, if you are born in the *day*, (Sun above the horizon); while Saturn is *also* above the horizon; *and* simultaneously posited in a masculine sign (Aries, Leo, Sagittarius, Gemini, Libra, Aquarius), then he is in a positive condition termed "Hayze". This fortunate condition warms up Saturn and renders him less pathologically cold/slow upon the body. Saturn in Hayze is still capable of indicating structural problems but less likely to produce diseases resultant from poor circulation and/or the obstruction of the vital force.

   Study the body areas ruled by the sign Saturn tenants in the birth chart. What conditions might manifest if these bodily parts are impeded, chilled, restricted? The lists below will lend ideas, but this list is only partial at best. You must learn to do this yourself! Just think of the words "cold, impaired, obstructed, deposits or structural issues" as applied to any of the body parts in this list.

## SATURN'S PATHOLOGICAL EFFECTS ON THE INDICATED BODY PART:

Saturn "cools" the body part he tenants in the birth chart. He also casts his dark blue cooling rays on the signs opposite or 180° away from his natal position (most); and sometimes upon the signs squaring or 90° from his position. The backwards square of Saturn is most powerful. That is, the casting of his ray to the sign 90° previous.

*Note*: Below is a brief list of potential health issues indicated by Saturn's placement in each sign. *However, Saturn's position in a sign certainly does not mean that one suffer from all these maladies!* Apply what you know of Saturn's nature (above) to the body parts listed under each sign and you will get the feel of what conditions might result. Naturally, not all conditions listed are mandatorily attendant to Saturn in said sign.

## SATURN'S SIGN REFLEXES:

At the end of each section, "Reflexes to" means that Saturn's listed potential problems could "bounce" to a reflexing sign (square or opposed sign), or to a planet in said sign. This is most likely to occur should the other "planet" be the Sun, Moon or ruler of the ascendant, 6th, 8th or 12th houses. More importantly, "reflex to" means that Saturn will manifest through the problems of the sign he opposes, and (less often), squares, rather than the issue of the sign he is in. Saturn in reflex behaves as though he is posited the reflexing sign, rather than in the sign he really inhabits in the birth chart.

For instance, Saturn in Sagittarius might reflex to Gemini, thus manifesting as arm and hand problems rather than as the traditional Sagittarian hip and thigh issues. You might think of this as his throwing his cold ray on to the opposite sign, and sometimes to his squaring signs as well. I've listed the reflex signs always in order of strength of the reflex. The opposing sign first. The backward square aspect second. The forward square aspect is third in importance.

SATURN'S PATHOLOGICAL ACTION IN THE TWELVE SIGNS

*Note*: Natal Saturn in any of the signs does not insure you will have the conditions given below. Should your Saturn be afflicted by aspect, in detriment or fall, retrograde or in association with the 1st, 6th, 8th or 12th houses, or their planetary rulers, then possibly he may exhibit one or more of the listed complaints. He may do so anyway, being Saturn, but this is not guaranteed. He is better placed in the 6th and 8th than any of the other planets and if well aspected and dignified, may surprise you by producing good health when in "evil" houses!

SATURN IN ARIES: Restricts blood vessels of brain. Headaches, toothache, eyesight issues, motor nerve anomalies, skull anomalies, stroke, hardening of arteries in brain.
*Reflexes to*: Libra, Cancer, Capricorn. (see body parts they rule).

SATURN IN TAURUS: Restricts the ear, nose throat region. Toxic tonsils, chronic colds and sore throat, poor hearing, hypo thyroid, tight neck muscles, atlas bone out of place; structural restrictions of cervical vertebrae, TMJ, dental issues.
*Reflexes to*: Scorpio, Leo, Aquarius.

SATURN IN GEMINI: Stuttering, restriction to lung, arm or hand, asthma- the "cold" variety, pulmonary consumption, bronchitis. Arthritic arms, shoulders, hands. Frozen shoulder, cystic fibrosis, emphysema, pneumonia. *Reflexes to*: Sagittarius, Pisces, Virgo.

SATURN IN CANCER: Restricts the breasts, rib cage, stomach, womb, sensitive skin, weak tooth enamel, osteoporosis, fear. Insufficient milk, small breasts, low hydrochloric acid, poor appetite, small chest, infertility, weak eyes, senility, low libido (effects hormones), dry mucous membrane, poor gums, drowning, falling, weak lungs, pneumonia, phobia.
*Reflects to:* Capricorn, Libra, Aries.

SATURN IN LEO: Restricts the heart muscle and stiffens the back: Heart attack, spinal anomaly, spinal cord disease, sclerosis of spinal cord, scoliosis, blood pressure extremes. Gives great strength in houses 1, 2, 3.
*Reflexes to:* Aquarius, Taurus, Scorpio.

SATURN IN VIRGO: Hernia, toxic liver, cirrhosis of liver, diabetes, constipation, dry membrane of bowel, appendicitis (especially near 16-19°

Virgo, Scorpio or Near 23° Gemini); premature gray hair due to malabsorbtion of nutrients, tension, insomnia, hernia.
*Reflexes to:* Pisces, Gemini, Sagittarius.

SATURN IN LIBRA: Mineral deposits in small tubules of kidneys, gravel, retention of urine, hormonal under activity, tension in lower back, Bright's disease.
*Reflexes to:* Aries, Capricorn and Cancer.

SATURN IN SCORPIO: Sterility, impotence, sexual issues, venereal disease, parasites, Crohn's disease, plugged sweat glands (sudoriferous glands), hemorrhoids, hernia, constipation, sluggish or toxic colon, amennorrhea, poisoning, gout, fractured pelvis, insufficient peristalsis, prostate cancer or obstruction.
*Reflexes to:* Taurus (look for gravel voice or throat ailments as a clue to a toxic colon), Leo, Aquarius.

SATURN IN SAGITTARIUS: Spinal misalignment, spinal cord diseases, arthritis of hips, hip and thigh problems; pressure on sciatic nerve, fractured pelvis.
*Reflexes to:* Gemini, Virgo, Pisces.

SATURN IN CAPRICORN: Skin issues - warts, dryness, cancer sensitivity, liver spots, skin disease. Infertility. Rheumatic knees, toxic liver, plugged gall ducts, insufficient bile, brittle nails, cuticle, teeth and gum issues, knee injuries, "ashy" skin and pigmentation anomalies. Falling.
*Reflexes to*: Cancer, Libra, Aries.

SATURN IN AQUARIUS: Broken ankle, obstructed circulation, low blood pressure, cold extremities, insufficient oxygenation of the blood, asthenia, pernicious anemia, hypothermia. Back issues, weak heart (opposes Leo).
*Reflexes to:* Leo, Taurus, Scorpio.

SATURN IN PISCES: Bad feet, corns, bunions, weak immunity, lung weakness (reflex from Gemini), wasting, apathy, depression, poor attention to health and diet, weak teeth, rickets, toxic or sluggish lymphatics, cold feet, calluses, corns.
*Reflexes to:* Virgo, Gemini, Sagittarius.

MARS, THE STIMULATOR

Mars, a traditional malefic, is the planet most implicated in acute illness. When afflicted or in excess, the sign of the body part he tenants may receive wounds, surgery, boils or display a scar, mole or freckle.

A Mars gone bad is too hot and red. An excess of heat and the color red is not good for the human body. By this very heated nature, Mars is the second "naturally" pathological planet and its position in the birth chart indicates an area for acute conditions. *See Also Mars' Associations, page 70.*

MARS RULES: Adrenaline, testosterone, male organs, the sense of smell, the catabolic metabolism (burning of fuel), the release of toxins, the red blood cells, iron, muscle tissue. The entire muscular system, inclusive of tendons and ligaments is under the rulership of Mars. Traditionally, Mars rules the left ear and Saturn the right. However, the ears are also generally under the rulership of Taurus and the sense of hearing is under Mercury.

PHYSICAL EFFECTS OF MARS: Stimulating, speeding up, inflaming, heating, breaking down, pushing out. Violent itching is also associated with some Mars conditions, especially when Mars is in Earth or Water signs.

Positive: Mars gives strength, courage, muscle tone, athletic prowess.

MARS' PATHOLOGICAL EFFECTS ON A GIVEN BODY PART

In excess, Mars heats up the body parts indicated by the natal or reflexing sign (below) to excess. Accidents, wounds, cuts and surgery are common to these areas.

Mars produces inflammation and expulsion. He is the great invader, thus indicated for all invasions of the bodily defenses by bacteria, virus or parasites, especially where symptoms include fever, rash, vomiting, diarrhea or blistering.

*SPECIAL CONDITIONS OF MARS: IMPORTANT!*

If you are *born in the day*, with (naturally) the Sun above the horizon; *and* your Mars is also above the horizon; *and* simultaneously posited in a masculine sign, then Mars is *extremely hot*. Mars in the above condition may manifest inflamed or overheated conditions in the bodily regions of his birth sign, or those in reflex. He must be watched closely, and if possible, antidoted. (The masculine signs are: Aries, Gemini, Leo, Libra, Sagittarius,

Aquarius. Aries, Leo and Sagittarius are the hottest!)

When so inflamed (day birth, above ground and in a masculine sign), he will throw off heat, speed up the metabolism and create rash, fever, irritation or other acute conditions related to the sign he is in or perhaps reflexing instead to the signs he squares, opposes or quincunxes. Cooling, demulcent and alterative herbs are useful. Any of of the three conditions above encourages Mars to overheat: (day birth, Mars above the horizon, and Mars in a masculine sign).

Conversely, a *night birth*, (Sun under the horizon); with Mars *simultaneously* under the horizon; and *also* Mars in the feminine signs (Taurus, Cancer, Virgo, Scorpio, Capricorn, Pisces); cools him off, and slows the metabolism. Less so in Scorpio. A cooler Mars position gives great endurance and internal strength. However a "too cool" Mars may have trouble ridding the body of waste or burning calories! A unnaturally chilly Mars is one of many astrological conditions contributing to obesity. Any one of the above three conditions above) will act to reduce the natural heat of Mars: (night birth, Mars under the horizon, Mars in feminine signs).

REFLEX ACTION OF MARS: Mars reflexes primarily to the the sign 90° ahead of it in zodiacal order. Secondarily Mars reflexes to the sign behind it by 90°; and also to the sign opposed, or 180° distant. The Vedic astrologers have discovered the backward "square" of Mars to not be as potent as the forward square, hence I list it as a secondary reflex. *The Vedic astrologers also report one of the strongest aspects of Mars to be its 8th house "quincunx" angle to another planet - a position 150° behind a planet in zodiacal order.* Personally, the author has seen the forward quincunx of Mars to also be effective. I will mention both signs that Quincunx each sign last under "reflexes", with the favored backward quincunx first).

WHAT DOES *REFLEX* MEAN IN MEDICAL ASTROLOGY?

First, Mars is able to heat up the three signs he reflexes to, and the two signs he quincunxes (as below). These signs can then behave (at times) as if Mars is in *them*, instead of the sign where he actually is!

This reflexive behavior of Mars' heating phenomenon primarily occurs if there is a planet in the sign that is posited in the either the reflexing or quincunxing signs in relation to the birth position of Mars. But this need not be the case! The sign receiving the rays of Mars by reflex or quincunx may be devoid of any planet and still produce Mars symptomology.

For example, Mars in Scorpio, the sign of the colon, might instead behave as if he were posited in Scorpio's opposite sign Taurus (rather than in Scorpio) and reflex as the astrological signification for tonsillitis. This can be explained by toxic build up in the colon (ruled by Scorpio) reflexing as infections in the throat area, which is governed by Taurus.

In searching a chart for the astralic source for a health problem - always start with the sign of the body part first, and then, study the reflex signs, and in the special case of Mars, his quincunxing signs too, listed here below.

MARS IN DIGNITY AND DEBILITY

Mars is more himself in his signs of *rulership* (Aries and Scorpio); makes good use of his energy in his sign of *exaltation* (Capricorn); is out of character in his signs of *detriment* (Libra and Taurus); and weak or malfunctioning in his *fall* (Cancer), a sign that forces his normally extroverted, assertive energy to become introverted and defensive.

Taurus, the detriment of Mars, does not weaken him. Far from it. Taurus being the sign of Mars' own North Node! One notices that individuals with Mars in Taurus may have a slow metabolism, but they possess unusual muscular strength, patience in work and notable endurance. They are hard workers and plenty assertive when necessary. Taurus merely alters the speedy and flammable nature of Mars by slowing him down and cooling him off.

Mars Rules: Aries and Scorpio
Mars Exaltation: Capricorn (best at 28°)
Mars Detriment: Libra and Taurus
Mars Fall: Cancer (peaks at 28°)

*Note*: Natal Mars in any of the signs does not insure one will have the conditions given below. Should your Mars be afflicted by aspect, in detriment or fall, retrograde or in association with the 1st, 6th, 8th or 12th houses, or their planetary rulers, then possibly he may exhibit one or more of the listed complaints. He may do so anyway, being Mars, but this is not guaranteed.

Mars is better placed in the 6th and 8th than any of the other planets except fellow malefic Saturn, and if well aspected and dignified, may surprise you by producing excellent health when in "evil" houses!

MARS' PATHOLOGICAL ACTION IN THE TWELVE SIGNS

MARS in ARIES: Dry hair, dry eyes, conjunctivitis, shooting pains in head, wounds to head and eyes, stroke, aneurism, capillary bleeding in brain, heatstroke, smallpox, brain fever, rosacea, measles, nosebleed, meningitis. People with Mars in this sign need to be very careful not to become too angry or allow their heads to become too hot. These folks run high, fast fevers, acne, wounds to head or eyes.
*Reflexes to*: Libra, Cancer, Capricorn.
*Quincunxes*: Scorpio, Virgo.

MARS IN TAURUS: Quinsy, sore throat, tonsillitis, strep throat, hyperthyroid, laryngitis, pharyngitis, injuries to ear, nose, throat, neck, venereal disease, thrush, herpes of mouth, acne (due to toxins in colon), wounds to neck or any Taurus region.
*Reflexes to:* Scorpio, Leo, Aquarius.
*Quincunxes:* Sagittarius, Libra.

MARS IN GEMINI: Asthma (hot variety), bronchitis. Pain in nerves of shoulders, arms and hands. Cuts to hands, neuritis, pleurisy, insomnia, overactive nerves, pneumonia.
*Reflexes to:* Sagittarius, Virgo, Pisces.
*Quincunxes:* Capricorn, Scorpio.

MARS IN CANCER: Acid stomach, ulcer, stomach flu, breast issues, infertility due to chemical imbalance of uterus, gastritis, irritated nipples, dyspepsia, pneumonia, wet inflammation of skin (poison oak type), stomach ulcer, boils, carbuncles, inflammation of mucous membrane, violent allergies, wounds to breast or stomach.
*Reflexes to:* Capricorn, Libra, Aries.
*Quincunx:* Aquarius, Sagittarius.

MARS IN LEO: Inflammation of heart, high blood pressure, back injury, inflammation of spinal cord, angina pectoris, aneurism, wounds to heart or back, dangerously high fevers, fevers that damage spinal cord.
*Reflexes to:* Aquarius, Scorpio, Taurus.
*Quincunxes:* Pisces, Capricorn.

MARS IN VIRGO: Diverticulitis, pancreatitis, diabetes (due to overwork of the pancreas), colitis, dry bowel, parasites, appendicitis (16-19° Virgo are related to the appendix), worms, intestinal flu, ventral hernia, allergies due to hyperactive immune response, insect bite reaction, wounds to abdomen.
*Reflexes to:* Pisces, Sagittarius, Gemini.
*Quincunxes:* Aries, Aquarius.

MARS IN LIBRA: Kidney infection, adrenal exhaustion, sex hormone imbalance, nephritis, pyelitis, acne (due to hormones), wounds to lower back or kidney.
*Reflexes to*: Aries, Capricorn, Cancer.
*Quincunxes*: Taurus, Pisces.

MARS IN SCORPIO: Vaginitis, mennoraghia, bladder infection, infection of female organs, nose bleed, uterine hemorrhage, miscarriage, abortion, venereal diseases, infection or injury of male organs, colitis, hemorrhoids, worms of the colon and anus, excess sex hormones, chronic diarrhea, acne (due to vigorous throwing off of toxins). Violent anal or genital itching. Waterborne diseases. Wounds to genitals or nose.
*Reflexes:* Taurus, Aquarius, Leo.
*Quincunxes:* Gemini, Aries.

MARS IN SAGITTARIUS: Sciatica, groin pulls, strain to hip, glutteal or thigh muscles, hyperactivity, insomnia, athletic injuries, enteric fever, gunshot wounds. The motor nerves seem greatly agitated by this position.
*Reflexes to:* Gemini, Pisces, Virgo.
*Quincunxes*: Cancer, Taurus.

MARS IN CAPRICORN: Knee injury, skin diseases of hot and/or dry quality: rash, itch, redness, heat. Erysipelas, psoriasis, measles, scabies, dry skin, carbuncles, boils, scars, keloids.
*Reflexes to*: Cancer, Aries, Libra.
*Quincunxes:* Leo, Gemini.

MARS IN AQUARIUS: Sprained ankles, blood poisoning, wounds to lower leg. Effects heart through reflex action to Leo.
*Reflexes to:* Leo, Taurus, Scorpio.
*Quincunxes:* Virgo, Cancer.

44

MARS IN PISCES: Restless feet syndrome, hot feet, foot injuries, toxic blood, lymphatic infection, mumps, duodenal ulcer, hyper sexuality, substance abuse, lung weakness, blood born diseases, poison oak, blisters, boils, blood parasites, waterborne disease, bleeding (difficulty clotting), foul body odor due to metabolic disorder.

*Reflexes to:* Virgo, Gemini, Sagittarius.

*Quincunxes:* Libra, Leo.

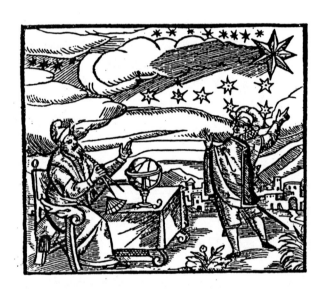

# The "Benefics" Venus and Jupiter.

Venus (the lesser benefic) and Jupiter (the greater) are noted for bringing protections, comforts and all good things. Nevertheless, when it comes to health they represent a type of energy flow just like any other planet. Venus being soft, sweet and atonic brings diseases of like nature. She excels in the ailments brought about by pleasure, neglect, sugar, parasitically inviting internal environments and soft muscular tone. She is prone to cysts, usually benign, and to candida albicans. She soothes pain.

One can always have too much of a good thing. Venusian people may be pretty, but they are rarely concerned about their health. However, Venus conditions are usually correctable and not life threatening.

Jupiter the Greater Benefic, brings growth. Expansion is good for your pocket book but not your waist size or blood pressure! Jupiter can prove a first rate malefic in regards to health, ruling a train of deadly diseases including diabetes, obesity, high blood pressure, large tumors and liver disease.

BENEFICS AND TUMOR GROWTH

Regarding "benefics", it has been repeatedly noted that conjunctions and trines between Venus and Jupiter, especially when occurring in Water or Earth signs, may encourage cyst and tumor growth, usually benign. This tendency is all the more marked should the Moon also be conjunct or trine a benefic. The fortunate nature of fertility and growth are relative!

VENUS THROUGH THE SIGNS: *See Venus Associations, page 70.*

These expressions of Venus are only a potential. Venus in any particular sign does not mean one has these conditions. IMPORTANT NOTE: Below we have listed Venus' pathologies. However, Venus is a benefic - the "lesser benefic" to be exact. *She brings beauty, magnetism and pleasure.*

If Venus is well aspected, we are likely to exhibit health and beauty in the areas mentioned! For example, as Venus in Aries often gives sparkly eyes and a pretty face! And Venus in Pisces gives nice feet or at least the desire to decorate them! Venus soothes and comforts. She is magnetic.

The pathological expressions of Venus are rare. To indicate disease, Venus must be poorly aspected, and/or in *debility* i.e. her *detriment* or *fall* positions, below. She performs best in *rulership* and *exaltation*. See *Note*.

VENUS IN DIGNITY AND DEBILITY
Venus Rules: Taurus and Libra
Venus Exalted: Pisces (best at 27°)
Venus Detriment: Scorpio and Aries
Venus Fall: Virgo (peaks at 27°)

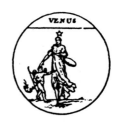

*Note*: Natal Venus in any of the signs does not ensure you will have the conditions given below. Should one's Venus be afflicted by aspect; in her signs of detriment or fall; retrograde or in association with the 1st, 6th, 8th or 12th houses, or their planetary rulers, then possibly she may exhibit one or more of the listed complaints. She can also assist any sign she tenants.

## VENUS' MEDICAL INFLUENCE IN THE TWELVE SIGNS

VENUS IN ARIES: Acne, female hormone issues, kidney complaints, ovarian problems. Sparkling eyes and attention - catching hair or face, premature baldness.

VENUS IN TAURUS: Problems due to gormandizing, slow thyroid, fatty buildup in neck vessels, weak neck. Catarrh in ear, nose and throat causing infection. Soft teeth, swellings of neck glands, excess saliva, vocal polyps. Sensual lips and lovely voice. Abundant hair (Taurus is less inclined to baldness then some other signs).

VENUS IN GEMINI: Weak lungs, raised lipid levels in blood, lack of muscular development in arms. Nice hands (or decorated hands and arms).

VENUS IN CANCER: Swelling breasts, cysts, obesity, beautiful breasts.

VENUS IN LEO: Lazy heart muscle, low blood pressure, weak back, enlarged heart, beautiful back.

VENUS IN VIRGO: Sluggish liver, intestinal worms, peristaltic debility, lazy bowel.

VENUS IN LIBRA: Insufficient kidney action, acne, alcoholism, excess love of sweets, anuria, fallopian pregnancy, fallopian tumor. Unusual beauty.

VENUS IN SCORPIO: Candida, yeast infection, excess sexual secretion, hemorrhoids, venereal disease, inguinal hernia, prolapsed uterus, uterine tumor, genital herpes, problems due to abortion or miscarriage, toxic colon, worms.

VENUS IN SAGITTARIUS: Soft hip bones, cysts in hip area. (Also gives pretty legs!)

VENUS IN CAPRICORN: Venus seems to benefit the skin in this sign. Skin eruptions may occur if ill aspected, because insufficient action of skin to expel toxins; or due to toxic buildup outletting through the skin (boils, carbuncles, warts, shingles, liver spots), plugged sweat or oil glands. Gout in knee area. Also, beautiful skin, pretty knees.

VENUS IN AQUARIUS: Varicose veins, weak ankles, low blood pressure or sluggish circulation, edema in lower legs.

VENUS IN PISCES: Foot blisters, excessive sex drive, glandular disorder, athlete's foot, fungus, high blood sugar. Also, nice feet.

## JUPITER THE EXPANSIVE _See Jupiter's Associations, page 70._

Jupiter is the _Greater Benefic_. However, he can also be a first rate indicator of a health pathology. How can this be? Ever heard of too much of a good thing? Jupiter gives too much: too much fat, too much blood, too much energy, too much heat - all depending on the sign he is in at birth. Remember, Jupiter rules fat, and excessive fat in any body part can also cause serious problems.

Jupiter is more likely to be productive of illness when in _debility_, i.e. his _detriment_ or _fall_ positions given below.

_Note:_ Jupiter's transits are less welcome for Virgo, Gemini and Capricorn ascendants, and can become a first rate _temporary malefic_ for birth charts with these ascendants unless brilliantly aspected and well placed in the natal chart.

Jupiter shares rulership of the liver with Virgo. The liver may become sluggish when Jupiter is in detriment. In reverse, Jupiter may produce excessive expansion in his signs of dignity, e.g. excessive circulating blood cholesterol when in Pisces, his sign of rulership.

JUPITER IN DIGNITY AND DEBILITY
Jupiter Rules: Pisces, Sagittarius
Jupiter Exalted: Cancer (best at 15°)
Jupiter Detriment: Virgo, Gemini
Jupiter Fall: Capricorn (peaks at 15°)

*Note*: Natal Jupiter in any of the signs does not insure you will have the conditions given below. Should your Jupiter be afflicted by aspect, in Detriment or Fall, retrograde or in association with the 1st, 6th, 8th or 12th houses, or their planetary rulers, then possibly he may exhibit one or more of the listed complaints.

## JUPITER'S PATHOLOGICAL INFLUENCE IN THE TWELVE SIGNS

JUPITER IN ARIES: Bursts of high blood pressure, excess blood to brain, headaches, thrombosis, vertigo, overactive motor centers, excess firing of any part of brain, epilepsy, strokes, hot flashes, overheating, brain tumor.

JUPITER IN TAURUS: Fatty neck vessels, tumors in throat, congestion in ear-nose-throat, sore throats, apoplexy, hypo thyroid, overeating. This position is prone to liver toxicity and congestion of the colon. Overgrowth of teeth. Vocal nodes, goiter. Abundant hair, or hirsute.

JUPITER IN GEMINI: Nervous scattering, pulmonary embolism, lung ailments, tumors in Gemini regions - lungs, hands, arms.

JUPITER IN CANCER: Excess breast tissue, mastitis, stomach and uterine growths, excess appetite leading to obesity, edema, torpid liver, bloating, stomach gas, breast tumors.

JUPITER IN LEO: Fatty degeneration of heart, heart attack, high blood pressure, enlarged heart, cerebral hemorrhage. Large torso.

JUPITER IN VIRGO: Overworked pancreas, jaundice, fatty degeneration of liver, intestinal growths.

JUPITER IN LIBRA: Poor venous circulation, fatty kidneys, hormonal disturbance, acne, ovarian and fallopian cysts or tumors.

JUPITER IN SCORPIO: Enlarged prostate, uterine fibroids, swollen testicles, difficulty holding urine, excessive perspiration, swollen nose, incontinence, involuntary ejaculation, hydremia, edema, excessive secretions of urates, excessive sex hormones, hirsuteness.

JUPITER IN SAGITTARIUS: Hyptertension, stroke, tumors in hips or thighs, obese lower body, pressure of growths upon sciatic nerve, religious grandiosity, insomnia, hyperactivity, gambling compulsions, madness, fatty buildup in arteries.

JUPITER IN CAPRICORN: Toxic liver, cirrhosis of liver, plugged gall ducts, skin ailments due to toxic condition of liver and/or disturbed sebaceous glands, jaundice, excema.

JUPITER IN AQUARIUS: Varicose veins, edema of ankles, weak heart action, leukemia, blood disorders, lumbago, disorders of the vessels of the lower leg, growths in lower legs.

JUPITER IN PISCES: Swollen glands, lymphatic disorders, high cholesterol in blood, excessive sex drive, large feet, swollen feet, glandular disturbance, obesity, dwarfism, growth disturbances, edema (especially in feet but anywhere), dropsy, iatrogenic diseases.

# The Nervous Planets: Mercury and Uranus

## MERCURY: THE MESSENGER

Mercury is a nervous planet, imparting a high strung quality to the body areas governed by the sign he tenants at birth. Omar Garrison notes in *Medical Astrology, How the Stars Influence Your Health,* that Mercury is able to change the direction and/or raise or lower the vibratory rate of the electromagnetic currents moving through the nerves and cells.

Mercury - a hermaphrodite in mythology - is the fastest moving planet. It makes good sense that he governs the speed of our neural synapses and how efficiently we receive and identify sense data through the afferent nerves. One might liken Mercury to a great communications switchboard between the internal and external environment. Mercury's effects are similar to Uranus, though potentially less serious and also easier to diagnose. *See Mercury's Associations, page 70.*

## MERCURY IN DIGNITY AND DEBILITY

Mercury is apt to act mentally muggier or careless in his *debility*, i.e. his signs of *detriment* and *fall*, below. However, if ill aspected, he becomes hyperactive and prone to nervous strain in his signs of dignity (i.e. *rulership* and *exaltation*).

<u>Mercury Rules:</u> Gemini and Virgo  (best at 15°)
<u>Mercury Exalted:</u> Aquarius
<u>Mercury Detriment:</u> Sagittarius and Pisces (peaks at 15° Pisces)
<u>Mercury Fall:</u> Leo, Sagittarius

*Note:* Natal Mercury in any of the signs does not insure you will have the conditions given below. Should your Mercury be afflicted by aspect, or in detriment or fall, or retrograde; or in association with the 1st, 6th, 8th or 12th houses, (or their planetary rulers), then possibly he may exhibit one or more of the listed complaints.

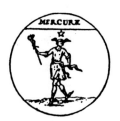

MERCURY'S PATHOLOGICAL EFFECTS IN THE TWELVE SIGNS

*Note*: Mercury's signs of reflex action are not included because of the limited aspect casting powers of this planet. However, if interested, you can use the same sign reflexes as given for Uranus.

MERCURY IN ARIES: Shooting pains in head, itchy eyes, head lice, neuralgia, facial ticks, nervous headache, nervous eyestrain, eye discoordination, astigmatism, misfiring signals in brain, overactive pineal, teeth sensitivity, epilepsy.

MERCURY IN TAURUS: Hearing loss, tinitus, teeth sensitivity, hoarseness, speech defects, dumbness, urinary incontinence, pains in ears, vocal anomalies.

MERCURY IN GEMINI: Stuttering, speech disorders, epilepsy, palsy in arms, carpal tunnel disorder, nervous pains in shoulders, arms, hands, nervousness, tremors, intercostal neuralgia, asthma, bronchitis, respiratory irritations.

MERCURY IN CANCER: Nervous stomach, sensitive breasts and nipples, mental disturbance, depression, nearsightedness, sensitive gums, emotions effect digestion, allergies, susceptibility to colds, weak upper lungs, stomach cramps, paranoia.

MERCURY IN LEO: Heart palpitation, neurological pains in back, contributing testimony toward diseases of the spinal cord, heart arrhythmia, malfunctions in heart valves.

MERCURY IN VIRGO: Nervous indigestion, hypochondria, colic, diarrhea, insomnia, anxiousness, neurosis.

MERCURY IN LIBRA: Dizziness, urinary incontinence, urinary suppression, a contributing testimony of renal problems, renal paroxysms, nervous headache, weak eyes.

MERCURY IN SCORPIO: Bladder irritation, painful urination, itching genitals, itching anus, worms, colon and rectal parasites, lice, herpes, genital warts, incontinence, spastic colon, a contributing testimony of menstrual troubles, blood worm, depression.

MERCURY IN SAGITTARIUS: Sciatica, neural pains in hips and thighs, schizophrenia, insomnia, restlessness, nervous disorders.

MERCURY IN CAPRICORN: Itchy skin, intolerance of insect bites, pruritis, anxiety, nervous stomach, sensitive teeth, poor hearing, depression, overwork, neural pains in the knees, unstable knee.

MERCURY IN AQUARIUS: High - strung, neural pains in ankles, shooting pains anywhere in body, muscle cramps, disturbances to the electrical currents in the body, mental disorders, diseases involving the nerve fluids, sensitivity to electromagnetic fields and computers, a contributing testimony to circulatory disorders, cardiac arrhythmia.

MERCURY IN PISCES: Sensitive feet, neurological pains in feet, lung weakness, tuberculosis, pneumonia, depression, pthisis, amnesia, chilblains, hallucination, speech problems, mental confusion.

## URANUS THE ELECTRIC

URANUS: This planet rules *extremes*. His general action upon the body is to throw off necessary balances and/or disturb normal rhythm.

Astronomically speaking, Uranus rotates backward, lies on its side and possesses a reversed magnetic field when compared to the other planets. In the body, Uranus produces unexpected reverses of balances, spasms, thyroid disturbance and "undiagnosable" conditions related to electromagnetic currents.

Electricity is under the rulership of Uranus although Mercury is involved when assessing the general flow of current through the nerves and synapses. When Uranus is afflicted always consider an electrical disturbance as causative should the body parts governed by either the birth sign or transiting sign of Uranus be those afflicted. You may also consider the body parts governed by the signs square (90°) and opposing (180°) Uranus.

*Note*: Uranus at birth in any of the signs below does not insure or suggest you suffer from any of the below listed conditions. A seriously afflicted Uranus posited especially, but not necessarily in the 1st, 6th, 8th or 12th houses, may potentially, but not absolutely, outlet in one or more of these pathologies, or similar conditions not listed.
*See Uranus' Actions and Associations, page 71.*

URANUS' PATHOLOGICAL ACTION IN THE TWELVE SIGNS

URANUS IN ARIES: Epilepsy, facial paralysis, violent fits, inexplicable explosive rages, Tourette's syndrome, shooting pains in eyes or head, hyperactivity, stroke, sudden aneurism bursts, hyperactive centers in brain, sleep walking, neuralgia, meningitis, tinitus, hearing loss through explosion or sneezing, blood vessels bursting in eye, sudden blindness, shock, brain trauma, concussion.
*Reflexes to:* Libra, Cancer, Capricorn.

URANUS IN TAURUS: Thyroid disorders, hearing anomaly, tinitus, vocal cord anomaly, atlas bone and cervical displacement,TNJ, glandular disorder, weird dental problems.
*Reflexes to:* Scorpio, Leo, Aquarius.

URANUS IN GEMINI: Tremors, neurological disease, spasmodic asthma, schizophrenia, mental illness, asphyxia, nervous hands, stuttering, Tourrette's syndrome, tinitus, nervous break down, dislocated shoulder, frozen shoulder.
*Reflexes to*: Sagittarius, Virgo, Pisces.

URANUS IN CANCER: Stomach spasms, intermittent breast swelling, flatulence, emotional shock, hiccough, misaligned elbow, hypothermia, glandular and temperature extremes, miscarriage, eating disorders, anorexia, bulimia, rare genetic diseases, forgetfulness, falls, incoordination, paranoia, dislocated elbow.
*Reflexes to:* Capricorn, Libra, Aries.

URANUS IN LEO: Heart attack, electrical disturbances of heart, spinal anomaly, polio, hypertension, malfunction of heart valves, sunstroke.
*Reflexes to*: Aquarius, Taurus, Scorpio.

URANUS IN VIRGO: Intestinal spasm, ruptured appendix, hyper immune response resulting in allergies. Blood sugar swings.
*Reflexes to:* Pisces, Gemini, Sagittarius.

URANUS IN LIBRA: Renal spasm, urinary incontinence, premature ejaculation, venereal skin rash, disrupts balances of the sex hormones, inconsistent menses, dizziness, migraine (reflex to Aries).
*Reflexes to:* Aries, Cancer, Capricorn.

URANUS IS SCORPIO: Bladder spasm, urinary incontinence, premature ejaculation, disrupts sex hormones, spastic colon, genital aberrations, hermaphrodism, miscarriage, abortion, displaced sacrum or coccyx, genetic diseases.
*Reflexes to:* Taurus, Aquarius, Leo.

URANUS IN SAGITTARIUS: Sciatica, St. Vitus' dance, serious neurological illness, misfiring of motor nerves, insanity, schizophrenia, insomnia, sleep walking, accidents to hip and thigh, spasm in hip and thigh, hyperactivity, hallucination, muscle spasm. Accidents due to sports, horses, driving, war or hunting. Dislocated hips, spinal anomaly.
*Reflexes to:* Gemini, Virgo, Pisces.

URANUS IN CAPRICORN: Trick knee, neuralgia, tetanus (?- O. Garrison), sudden outbreaks of skin rash or eruption, rare skin diseases, stomach spasm, eating disorders, anorexia, bulimia, rare genetic diseases, falls, rare bone diseases, disruptions of mineral balances in body and bone, oddities of bone growth or structure, osteoporosis, dementia, miscarriage, infertility.
*Reflexes to:* Cancer, Aries, Libra.

URANUS IN AQUARIUS: Electrical system in body becomes erratic, muscle spasm, circulatory irregularity, inexplicable spasms and shooting pains, nervous, nightmares, leg spasms, electrocution, shock, nervous break down, rare diseases of nervous system or blood, heart palpitation, disruption of heart rhythm, sickle cell anemia.
*Reflexes to:* Leo, Scorpio, Leo.

URANUS IN PISCES: Restless foot syndrome, structural anomaly of feet, rare blood disorders, claustrophobia, spastic asthma, galloping pneumonia, foot cramps, intense or disturbing dream life, hearing voices, glandular extremes influencing weight and growth, dwarfism, gigantism.
*Reflexes to:* Virgo, Gemini, Sagittarius.

# Neptune: the Dissolver

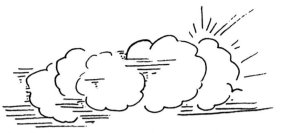

Neptune diffuses the energy of the body parts governed by the sign he tenants. His influence is draining, weakening and leaking. Magnetism is under his rule (with Venus) and therefore, he is implicated in cases of electromagnetic related fatigue. Conditions resultant from psychic draining are under his province.

Neptune's domain includes: gas leaks, viruses, hidden poisons, contagious illness and psychic suggestion, hypnosis, fatigue, sleeping. Neptune is the planet of sleep and his transits to important planets produce drowsiness. He confuses and clouds any issue, making correct diagnosis problematic. _See Neptune's Associations, page 71._

*Note:* Natal Neptune in any of the signs does not guarantee the health issues listed below. An afflicted Neptune, especially if posited in the 1st, 6th, 8th or 12th houses is more likely to produce one or more of the given complaints.

## NEPTUNE'S PATHOLOGICAL INFLUENCE
## IN THE TWELVE SIGNS

NEPTUNE IN ARIES: Weak eyes, blindness, cataract, brain tumor, excess sleep, drug and alcohol addiction (with Mars, South Node), blood poisoning (with Mars), gas poisoning, delusion, disorders of the cerebral ventricles, cerebral palsy.
*Reflexes to:* Libra, Cancer and Capricorn.

NEPTUNE IN TAURUS: Hearing disorders (or very sensitive ears), clairaudience, hypo thyroid, food cravings, polyps in vocal cords, accidental asphyxiation, cancer of mouth or esophagus, tooth decay.
*Reflexes to:* Scorpio, Leo, Aquarius.

NEPTUNE IN GEMINI: Water in lung, susceptablity to colds, weak chest, atrophy of arms, absent mindedness, addiction to smoked substances, poor lung action, hole in lung, lung tumor, shadows on lung, consumption, schizophrenia.
*Reflexes to:* Sagittarius, Pisces, Virgo.

NEPTUNE IN CANCER: Weak lungs, chest colds, poor immunity, weak stomach, sensitive breasts, tooth decay, fearfulness, nearsightedness, cataracts, breast tumors, photographic memory for past events but absent minded in present, excess weeping, fungus and mold problems, danger of drowning, fatigue.
*Reflexes to:* Capricorn, Aries, Libra.

NEPTUNE IN LEO: Weak heart muscle, low blood pressure, weak back, poor vision, blindness, cataracts, slipped intervertabrael discs, lax action of depressor nerve of heart, leaky heart valves or hole in heart, alcohol and drug effects to heart, grandiosity.
*Reflexes to:* Aquarius, Taurus, Scorpio.

NEPTUNE IN VIRGO: Leaky gut syndrome, toxic or under active liver, poor peristalsis, lazy colon, candida, hypochondria, liver flukes, obsessive compulsive disorder (OCD), toxic appendix build up, strange allergies, eating neurosis.
*Reflexes to:* Pisces, Gemini, Sagittarius.

NEPTUNE IN LIBRA: Insufficient kidney function, low kidney energy, leaky urine or semen, bed wetting, lethargy, fantasy addiction. Sugar, music or wine addiction. Sex and love addiction, music and movie addiction, gender identity disorder.
*Reflexes to:* Aries, Capricorn, Cancer.

NEPTUNE IN SCORPIO: Uterine fibroids, mennoraghia, anemia due to mennoraghia, spirit possession, effects of hypnotic control or black magic, parasites, candida and molds, vaginal yeast, jock itch, polyps in colon and rectum, hemorrhoids, sexual obsession or perversion, nymphomania, waterborne parasites of colon, STDs, herpes, AIDS, drug addictions.
*Reflexes to:* Taurus, Leo, Aquarius.

NEPTUNE IN SAGITTARIUS: Wanderlust, sleep walking, atrophy of hip and leg muscles, multiple sclerosis, religious ecstasy, insanity, palsy, peculiar disorders of nervous system and spinal cord, weakens lungs, arterial insufficiency or leak.
*Reflexes to:* Gemini, Pisces, Virgo.

NEPTUNE IN CAPRICORN: Weak knees, melanoma, moles, warts, fungus under nails, weak nails, tooth decay, insufficient mineral absorption in

*Neptune in Capricorn continued*
bones, malnutrition, wasting, rickets, pineal hypoplasia.
*Reflexes to:* Cancer, Libra, Aries.

NEPTUNE IN AQUARIUS: Sprained ankles, varicose veins, insufficient circulation, weak heart, leaks in heart valves, anemia, asexuality, gender identity disorder, low blood pressure, rare blood diseases, psychosis, alcoholism - last 5 degrees of sign implicated.
*Reflexes to:* Leo, Taurus, Scorpio.

NEPTUNE IN PISCES: Excess sleeping, flat foot, weak feet, athlete's foot, toe fungus, poisoned blood, rare blood diseases, lymphatic cysts, poor drainage of lymphatics, weak immune system and susceptibility to contagious illness. Pneumonia, tuberculosis, retardation, spirit possession, susceptibility to hypnotic control and suggestion. Mental delusions, fantasy, nymphomania, poor clotting, suicidal tendency.
*Reflexes to:* Virgo, Gemini, Sagittarius.

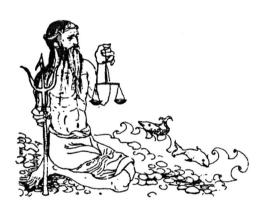

# Pluto, the Cathartic

Pluto and his health effects have not yet been observed through the twelve signs. This tiny, mustard colored "planet" (currently in question as such), was first discovered in 1930, in Cancer. At the time of this writing he is transiting through late Sagittarius, less than half way through the signs since his first observation by humans. We have seventy some years of written opinion on Pluto's recently observed effects, and at best, this is nascent research.

A great many writers have reiterated and developed the themes and character of the Greek god Pluto, the planet's obvious namesake. Their writings now largely establish the "traditional" meanings of Pluto. Opinions are only rarely backed by cited research, (requiring a minimum of of one hundred carefully documented personal case studies, replicated).

The author does not follow the unquestioned modern astrological doctrine that a planet's given name is therefore identical with his/her character via the mythological association. For instance, it has been pointed out by Richard Idemon, that Uranus would have been far more aptly named "Prometheus" because the Promethean mythological associations are truly a better fit than those of the namesake god Uranus.

Other writers have gifted Pluto the rulership over Scorpio and allotted him all the traditional associations with Mars, who enjoyed these privileges unquestioned for over two thousand years! Someone decided early on that Pluto should take over the rulership of Scorpio, instead of Mars, because Pluto sort of fit the sign (because of his name?) and well, gosh darn it, he needs a sign! Other contenders for Pluto's rulership might have been earthy and sensual Taurus (Pluto lived in the earth, hoarded wealth, and was notably sexy); or perhaps Leo, a willful sign sharing some of the powerful, drastic and volcanic qualities noted for Pluto. Cancer is Pluto's sign of discovery and also home of his North Node - so what is this Cancer-Pluto connection about? Certainly, it must mean something.

But why do the outer planets need to "rule" any sign? Let us observe them for a long time before assigning rulerships, if they are required at all. And let us think deeply about deposing Mars from his eons long reign over Scorpio, his night house.

In defining Pluto's rulerships based on the mythological Pluto namesake alone, we do a disservice to observation as first principal. Let us keep an open mind and observe Pluto's health effects for ourselves.

## POSSIBLE EFFECTS OF PLUTO

Pluto *may* relate to very serious or terminal conditions that demand the utmost application of the spiritual will. His transit is immensely powerful within an orb of 0-1° and may be negligible otherwise.

Edgar Cayce, the great medical psychic noted that not all people are receptive to Pluto, but that his effects were growing since the time of his discovery in the 1930s. The noted physicist Arthur Young (author of *The Geometry of Meaning* and *The Reflexive Universe,* and developer of the Bell helicopter), imparted to me his observation that few aspects were more powerful than transit Pluto's exact conjunction of a natal position.

Physicist Buryl Payne has linked Pluto in weather studies to extremely cold conditions. Other writers say he rules intense heat. It has been my observation that individuals born with Pluto closely rising, may emotionally blow hot or chill cold - my files suggest this planet rising at birth appears to be productive of unbending emotional extremes, autonomy and outstanding physical courage.

The author has witnessed him prominent (either by transit to the natal planets or under transit by them in the natal chart) at times of major life changing spiritual decisions, e.g. "I must stop smoking".

We all possess a gratification - seeking, survival oriented *animal will,* under Mars. This animal will is obvious throughout all of nature.
What planet reflects *the spiritual will,* that conscious direction of our life, controlling and disciplining this animal will? Some say Sol is "will", although he may reflect more the strength of the individuality and sense of purpose. *Perhaps the spiritual will has something to do with the mysterious little planet Pluto?*

In a study of rediscovery moments for sunken ships, I noted that Pluto would often cross a significant degree of the shipwreck chart. He seems to reveal that which is hidden, and to bring up that which lurks in the depths. You see, his mythological association may have something to it after all, but we must keep checking this out!

### PLUTO'S PATHOLOGY

Writers have speculatively linked Pluto pathologically with radiation, parasites, necrosis, cancer, cellular mutation, genetic problems, organ transplants, genetic conditions, drug detoxification programs, resistant bacteria, mysterious war - related poisonings, DNA and RNA, nucleic acid, retroviruses, enzymes, and severe poisoning from chemical or nuclear waste (this is likely as he was discovered during the development of the atomic bomb.) Pluto is also associated with obsession, possession, mass death and horrifying plagues. There is an agreement that he involves drastic conditions that demand an application of extreme methods and/or the absolute resolve of the spiritual will. *We see that Pluto shares many pathological assignments with Saturn, Mars and/or the Lunar South Node.*

Pluto's positive side may correlate him with amazing advances in genetics, transplants, limb regeneration as well as new methods for fighting viral and bacterial infection and plague control.

I will not attempt to list Pluto's affects in the twelve signs. It is enough to state that Pluto's health effects in any sign, *if negative* would be very serious indeed and associated with some of the issues noted above, such as the effects of nuclear radiation.

Personally, I've not witnessed Pluto *consistently* producing pathological effects in the signs - testifying to Edgar Cayce's idea that not all people were Pluto sensitive, and that his effect upon humanity is growing. Often, the bodily regions correlated with the sign of the natal Pluto appear in perfect health well into old age! Check this out in the birth charts of your friends and see what you find.

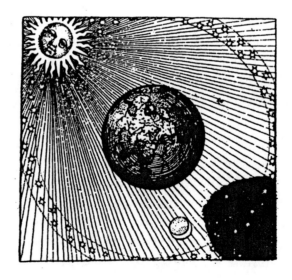

# The Lunar Nodes: Excess and Deficiency

The South Lunar Node (aka: Dragon's Tail, Ketu, Caput) is one of the three most important pathological points in the natal chart. The two others are Saturn and Mars.

The South Node always stands exactly *opposite* the North Node and their pathological action is indeed opposite. The Dragon's Tail represents the point where cosmic energy exits. The Dragon's Head is where cosmic energy enters. Think of a giant celestial pump, with energy being pumped into our sphere at the North Node and being defecated at the South Node. The Dragon's Head is where we have power "surges", or excess. Power outages occur at the Dragon's Tail, our potential point of deficiency and weakness.

The Tail is thus the great anus of the solar system from the perspective of the astrological health chart. Eclipses near this point signify a power outage, i.e. an exit or depletion of energy.

Planets closely conjoined this point are all too often impaired or gravely weakened. This is not always the case, but go find a planet in close conjunction with the Dragon's Tail, in a sign of it's detriment or fall; then throw in two or three afflicting aspects, and you will find a first rate problem of a kind related to the conjoining planet. One case from the files was of a woman with a retrograde Mars (surgery) in Libra (kidneys) conjunct the South Node. Her kidney was removed. A second example was of a boy with Mars in Taurus exactly conjoined the Tail who lost one testicle.

How does the "exit point" translate into one's health chart? Possibly, the sign and/or house placement of the South Node in your chart will signal a weak link in your anatomy. A pranic leak may be evident, perhaps a deficiency. *See South Node's Action and Associations, page 72.*

### South Node's Medical Associations:

Mental problems, parasites and molds, dirty conditions, and problems brought on by hypnosis, spirit possession, paranoia, gangrene, sepsis, poisons or black magic, and sometimes cancer, a disease more noted at the North Node.

You will find the draining influence similar to that of Neptune. Both points are weakening, sensitizing and psychically oriented. The oppositely positioned North Node is more cancer prone than the South Node, although the South Node can certainly be involved in certain cancers.

Hereditary conditions begotten from the parents are associated with both Lunar Nodes. Transiting planets crossing the South Node can indicate the onset of disease.

*Note:* A Natal position of your South Node in any of the signs does not guarantee you will have any of the cited conditions. Should your South Node be posited in the 1st, 6th, 8th or 12th, and squaring or conjoining a planet, or conjoined the planetary ruler of the above houses, then it is more likely to be productive of one or more of the listed conditions.

*Reflexes:* The Lunar Nodes cast no rays.

## THE SOUTH NODE'S PATHOLOGICAL ACTION IN THE SIGNS

SOUTH NODE IN ARIES: Weak eyesight, blindness, insufficient brain development, dropped on head as baby, weak upper teeth, weak blood vessels in brain, soft scull.

SOUTH NODE IN TAURUS: Poor hearing, harms self through diet, tooth decay, hypo thyroid, insufficient saliva, weak voice, food addictions.

SOUTH NODE IN GEMINI: Mental problems, insanity, epilepsy, weak arms, insufficient lung capacity, sensitive respiratory system, lost fingers, speech impediments.

SOUTH NODE IN CANCER: Weak stomach, sensitive breasts, infertility, paranoia of pregnancy, phobias in general, depression, mother fixations, miscarriage. Genetic conditions. Diseases arising from home, bed or bath environment. Environmental toxins, thin mucous membrane, weak uterine wall, insufficient milk.

SOUTH NODE IN LEO: Weakness in heart, weakness in back, weak eyesight.

SOUTH NODE IN VIRGO: Sluggish liver, pancreatic insufficiency, blood sugar problems, intestinal parasites, dystentery, diarrhea, hypochondria.

SOUTH NODE IN LIBRA: Insufficient kidney action, one kidney, hormonal disturbance, sugar addiction.

SOUTH NODE IN SCORPIO: Sexual insufficiency or alternatively addiction, depression, obsession, parasites or worms in colon, diarrhea, candida, vaginal yeast, jock itch, poisoning, great danger from blood transfusions or surgery, miscarriage, sepsis.

SOUTH NODE IN SAGITTARIUS: Weakness in hips or legs, neuromuscular diseases, arterial insufficiency, accidents through careless risk, drunk driving, jet lag.

SOUTH NODE IN CAPRICORN: Sensitive skin, weak knees, poor posture, career failures that may effect health, warts, moles, genetic conditions, mineral deficiency, osteoporosis.

SOUTH NODE IN AQUARIUS: Venous insufficiency, poor circulation, effects blood pressure (too high or low), weak ankles, edema, anemia.

SOUTH NODE IN PISCES: Weak feet, missing toes, foot and shoe problems, addictions, possession, hypnosis, susceptibility to contagious disease (weak immune system). Excessively responsive to psychic suggestion. Poisons in blood and lymph. Parasites or virus in blood or lymph. Depression, delusion, addiction.

## SOUTH NODE CONJUNCT THE PLANETS AND SIGNS

SOUTH NODE CONJUNCT SUN: Weak heart, low vitality, weak eye or blindness.

SOUTH NODE CONJUNCT THE MOON: Dysmennorhia, dehydration, malnourishment, infertility, insufficient milk, poor memory, depression, suicidal tendency.

SOUTH NODE CONJUNCT MERCURY: Speech impediments, hearing problems, weak arms, missing finger, paralysis, wasting of upper body, weak lungs, irrational thinking.

SOUTH NODE CONJUNCT VENUS: Blood sugar problems, wine, sugar or sex addiction, insufficient semen, weak skin, baldness, a psychological complex about one's appearance. Insufficiency of a female hormone.

SOUTH NODE CONJUNCT MARS: Anemia (low iron), sex addiction or avoidance (an extreme), accident prone, great danger in war or surgery, male erectile issues, karmic issues with male organs, tendency to vasectomy. Insufficiency of a male hormone, adrenal exhaustion.

SOUTH NODE CONJUNCT JUPITER: Insufficient fatty acids in blood, emaciation, poor liver function, insufficient growth hormone, growth disturbance, pituitary insufficiency, diabetes.

SOUTH NODE CONJUNCT SATURN: Osteoporosis, week teeth, malnutrition, mineral depletion, rickets, insufficient sexual development (Edgar Cayce says Saturn rules the gonads), bone disease, premature skin wrinkles, weak or blemished skin.

URANUS CONJUNCT SOUTH NODE: Insufficient electrical impulses in body, paralysis and atrophy due to lack of electrical current in nerve and muscle, spasms and cramps, power "outages" and "black- outs" in areas of body afflicted, mental aberrations. Great care should be taken with electrical appliances and lightning.

NEPTUNE CONJUNCT SOUTH NODE: Psychic disorders, potential double debility or weakness in area of body indicated in birth chart, pranic "leaks", atonic conditions, serious addictions, depression, lack of will power, tendency to suicide, past life memory hangovers upsetting the acceptance of present incarnation, danger of drowning. Drug overdose. Alcohol and drugs are "undoing"!

SOUTH NODE CONJUNCT PLUTO: Uncertain. Possibly rare genetic conditions, poisonings, parasites, bacteria, spirit possession, paranoia, gangrene, sepsis.


## THE NORTH NODE'S PATHOLOGICAL ACTION IN THE SIGNS

The North Lunar Node can sometimes contribute to a health condition, but not always. It can also suggest an an area of the body where we enjoy unusual strength. Alternative names for the North Node are: The Dragon's Head, Rahu and Caput.

Celestial energy enters at the Dragon's Head. Sometimes it enters too fast or too much. One often witnesses an excess of energy building up in the body parts of the sign the Head tenants at birth.

This point, representing the head of a greedy demon in mythology, ravenously gobbles up what is in his path. He is associated with cancer, addictions and skin diseases. Could serious autoimmune diseases in which the immune system attacks itself be related to the Dragon's Head? This area of inquiry is wide open.

Any natal planet in conjunction with this point is strongly placed. One will receive a lot of this planet's energy, but possibly too much, creating an imbalance. Below is a brief suggestive list of problems that might be associated with the Lunar North Node in each of the twelve signs. Ketu's influence is not unlike that of Saturn with a twinge of Pluto.
*See the North Node's Action and Associations, page 72.*

***The North Node's Medical Associations:***

He tends to produce growths, chronic and invasive conditions, toxic buildups, arthritic and rheumatic complaints, thickening and hardening. Together with the South Node, he governs inherited diseases.

Certain conditions can be related to either Node, due to the fact that they are always exactly opposite one another. However there are subtle differences in the underlying reasons for these same conditions. The Dragon's Head behaves with a will, and his pathological action is more deliberately aggressive and self - seeking. The Tail of the Dragon, having no "head", acts unconsciously.

Both Nodes are compulsive in behavior, and intense. However, the Head is more the aggressor and the Tail plays the victim. Example: South Node in Scorpio would be typical of a tendency to miscarry whereas North Node in Scorpio would-be more typical of abortion.

The transits of any planets over the Lunar North Node are extremely important because a lot of the transiting planet's energy will currently enter your life and body.

Both Lunar Nodes are associated with hereditary conditions begotten from the parents.

*Note:* A natal positioning of your North Node in any of the twelve signs does not guarantee you will have any of the cited conditions. Should your North Node be posited in the 1st, 6th, 8th or 12th, and squaring or conjoining a planet, or conjoined the ruler of the above houses, then it is more likely to be productive of one or more of the listed conditions.

NORTH NODE IN ARIES: Too much blood to the head, pressure to eyes (glaucoma), temper fits, hot head, heat stroke, stroke, aneurism, wounds to head or eyes, burns. Brain tumor.

NORTH NODE IN TAURUS: Obstructed ears, mucous build up in eustachian tubes and throat, vocal cord polyps. Cancer of mouth, throat or esophagus. Clogged jugulars or caratoids, excess wax build up in ears, hyperthyroid (?), food addictions, tooth decay, impacted wisdom teeth.

NORTH NODE IN GEMINI: Strong arms and hands, stiffening in arms, cystic fibrosis, lung cancer.

NORTH NODE IN CANCER: Breast tumors, stomach cancer, uterine fibroids.

NORTH NODE IN LEO: Hardening of vessels in heart, heart attack, strong back, lumbago, danger to heart from steroids, structural deformity of spine, disease of spinal cord.

NORTH NODE IN VIRGO: Intestinal growths, liver or pancreatic cancers, hyperactive immune reaction, allergies.

NORTH NODE IN KIDNEY: Sclerotic kidney, kidney stone, gout, toxemia, lumbago.

NORTH NODE IN SCORPIO: Uterine fibroid, problems from Viagra, thickening of vaginal wall, testicular cancer, prostrate cancer, bladder cancer, gout, gravel, toxemia, contagious blood or waterborne disease, abortion, excessive sex hormones, impacted sweat glands, broken nose.

NORTH NODE IN SAGITTARIUS: Growths in hip region, hardening of arteries. Hyperactive central nervous system, sciatica, structural deformity of hips or legs, neuromuscular diseases.

NORTH NODE IN CAPRICORN: Leprosy, excema, skin diseases, melanoma, warts, moles (conversely good skin), rheumatism of knees, heavy metal poisoning (especially lead).

NORTH NODE IN AQUARIUS: Effects blood pressure (high or low), strong ankles, weird blood diseases.

NORTH NODE IN PISCES: Corns, bunions, foot deformity, arthritis of feet, toxins in blood, lymphatic cancer, lymphatic swellings, autoimmune diseases (?), contagious blood born disease.

# NORTH NODE CONJUNCT THE PLANETS AND LIGHTS

NORTH NODE CONJUNCT SUN: Strong heart, high vital force, good vision, will. Big ego. Strength. One testimony of long life.

NORTH NODE CONJUNCT MOON: Large breasts, edema, dropsy, uterine fibroid. Excellent memory, fertile. Popularity with females. Successful wife. Excellent for vocations ruled by Moon.

NORTH NODE CONJUNCT MERCURY: Mercury poisoning, hardening of bones in ears. Also gives talent, elocution, writing ability and intelligence. Excellent for all vocations ruled by Mercury.

NORTH NODE CONJUNCT VENUS: Prone to soft benign cysts, sugar addiction, sex addiction, skin disease, moles, warts. (Also bestows beauty, charismatic appeal and popularity. Excellent for all vocations governed by Venus.

NORTH NODE CONJUNCT MARS: Abundant energy, strong muscles, athleticism, excess testosterone or adrenaline, large nose. Nerves of steel and terrific courage. One testimony of success as a surgeon! May run high fevers. Care of overheating, overexertion, aneurism, stroke. Successful for all careers governed by Mars. Great talent for surgeons.

NORTH. NODE CONJUNCT JUPITER: Obesity, excess cholesterol in blood and/arteries, fatty degeneration of liver, toxic liver, liver cancer, tumor prone - usually benign. Causes excess growth or size in area indicated in the birth chart, disturbs growth hormones. (For matters besides health, this position is one of the best bringing great luck and success in the house and sign combination indicated at birth). Success in Jupiterian careers.

NORTH NODE CONJUNCT SATURN: Rheumatic and sclerotic conditions in the sign indicated, bone growth, mineral deposits, spurs. Serious skin conditions, lupus, leprosy, lead or heavy metals poisoning, cancer prone. Strong bones and teeth. Positive for all Saturn ruled careers.

NORTH NODE CONJUNCT URANUS: Receives excess electrical energy, or unpredictable "power surges" into the house and sign indicated at birth. Disturbed sleep, energy surges, peculiar urges, electrical shock, radiation poisoning, hyperthyroid. Massive spasm and cramp. Great care should be taken with lightning and electricity! Positive for Uranus ruled careers.

NORTH NODE CONJUNCT NEPTUNE: Tumor prone. Edema, poor lymphatic drainage, excessive fungus or mold growth, candida, alcoholism, drug addiction, cravings. Positive for Neptune ruled careers.

NORTH NODE CONJUNCT PLUTO: Inclination to parasites and radiation or chemical poisoning of cells and DNA. Cancer and leukemia prone. AIDS, blood transfusions. Very serious diseases of karmic origin. Demonic spirit possession, disorders arising from black magic attack, epidemics, bacterial invasion, leprosy and serious "devouring" diseases. Destruction to cells by radiation therapy and chemotherapy, nuclear medicine. Sadism.
(May be one testimony of organ transplants, grafting and transfusions.) Brings luck and talent to surgeons. Success to Plutonian careers.

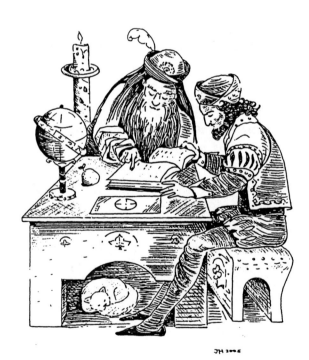

# Traditional Associations and Pathological Action of the Planets

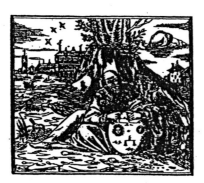

The foregoing chapters discussed in detail the medical effects of the two *lights* (Sun and Moon); *malefics* Saturn and Mars; *benefics* Venus and Jupiter; the nervous planets Mercury and Uranus; Lunar Nodes; Neptune; and Pluto.

For convenience rather than redundancy, the planets are listed again below, altogether, along with some new associations you might find useful.

## PLANETARY PATHOLOGY and ASSOCIATIONS

SUN: Rules Leo, Exalted in Aries.
*Action:* The battery of life force. Heating. The Sun emphasizes the sign he is in, and your vital force is qualified by this sign's quality more than by the sun's distinctive nature! What is meant by this? To explain, the Sun is hot and dry in energetic action, but you will not always see this drying effect in the body parts governed by the sign he tenants at birth. Instead, you may simply see an emphasis on the qualities and body parts of that sign, either positive or negative.
*Associations:* You may look to Sol's natal sign and house position to judge strength and burn rate of the natural vital force within the body. The Sun governs the Heart. This is very important to remember! Also, the right eye in the male and the left eye in the female. Gold. *See Chapters 2, 4.*

MOON: Rules Cancer, Exalted in Taurus. ☽

*Action:* Distributes the vital force of the Sun. Fluidic, changeable, sensitizing, reflexive, weakening, watery.

*Associations: Mammary glands, uterus, stomach, sympathetic nerves, colorless lymph (with Pisces), secreting functions, lungs (with Gemini for upper lobes of the lung and Cancer for the lober lobes).*

The mucous membranes. The right eye in the female and the left eye in the male. Silver. *See Chapter 5.*

MERCURY: Rules Gemini and Virgo. Exalted in Virgo and Aquarius. ☿

*Action:* Nervous, itchy. Mercury is the basic planet of the nerves.

*Associations:* The pineal gland (E. Cayce). Speech and hearing issues - check Mercury, sense of hearing and auditory nerves in general, sense of touch (with Venus), the tongue (with Taurus). The metal Mercury. *See Chapter 8.*

VENUS: Rules Taurus and Libra. Exalted in Pisces. ♀

*Action:* Sloppy, lazy, atonic. Pleasure - related problems, sugar. Venus (when negative) reduces muscular tone, and softens tissue.

*Associations:* female genitalia, skin, hair, the cheeks, lips and mouth, taste, touch (with Mercury), the ovaries, female hormones, semen, the womb (with Cancer and Scorpio). The thymus gland (Edgar Cayce). Venus possibly influence on thyroid gland (with Taurus and Uranus). Copper. *Chapter 7.*

MARS: Rules Aries and Scorpio. Exalted in Capricorn. ♂

*Action:* Heating, stimulating, inflaming, agitating, speeding, poisoning, throwing off, cutting, bleeding, wounding, invading, attacking (bacterial infection, aggressive parasites), violent itch.

*Associations:* The adrenal glands, adrenaline, the muscles, sense of smell, male hormones, virility, red blood corpuscles. General level of energy (combine with Sun). Iron.

*See Chapter 6.*

JUPITER: Rules Sagittarius and Pisces. Exalted in Cancer. ♃

*Action:* Expansive, fattening, growing (tumor prone), raises blood pressure in Fire signs.

*Associations:* Influences the arterial circulation (with Sagittarius). The liver in general (with Virgo). Fats. Carter points out that in accidents involving the legs in general, Jupiter is involved. This supports the link with Jupiter's sign Sagittarius, the sign which governs the hips and thighs. The pituitary gland (Edgar Cayce), the Isles of Langerhans. Tin. *Chapter 7.*

SATURN: Rules Capricorn and Aquarius. Exalted in Libra. ♄
*Action:* Freezing, depriving, limiting, restricting, concretizing, slowing, hardening, stiffening, strengthening, the gall and gall bladder.
*Associations:* The bones, cuticles, ligaments, skin, cuticles, nails, teeth (with Taurus), gall bladder. The gonads (Edgar Cayce). The strength of the body. Lead. Graphite. Calcium. *See Chapter 6.*

URANUS: Co-rules Aquarius with Saturn. Exalted in Gemini. ♅
*Action:* Uranus influences the electrical current in the body. Uranus gives spasm, sudden reversals, extremes, unforeseen surprise, chaos, imbalance to brain chemistry or hormones, and magnetic fields disturbances. Unpredictable effects may attend any major medical procedure during the days around a Uranus station, i.e. the days each year when Uranus changes direction when viewed from the earth. Uranus is prominent in the charts of transsexuals, especially in hard aspect to Mars or Venus. See also Neptune.
*Associations:* Uranus and Neptune relate to electromagnetic "poisoning". The motor nerves are associated with Uranus, Mars, Aries and Sagittarius. The thyroid gland (E. Cayce). Element: Uranium? *See Chapter 8.*

NEPTUNE: Co-rules Pisces with Jupiter. Exalted in Cancer. ♆
*Action:* Sedative, weakening, draining, confusing, lax functioning, clouding (wrong diagnosis).
*Associations:* Medically, Neptune governs secret poisoning, viruses, sedative drugs, candida type conditions, fungus, hypnotic states, suggestion, possession, magnetic radiation and its effect on the body. Electromagnetic poisoning. The spinal fluid (Cornell), sleep, endorphins. Neptune and/or Uranus in hard aspect to Mars and/or Venus may indicate gender identity disorder (GID). *See Chapter 9.*

PLUTO: Co-Rules Scorpio. ♇, ♀
*Action:* The jury still out on the "true" influence of Pluto (see theories, under Chapter 10). Pluto appears to intensify issues, and is noted for stimulating extremes of temperature: boiling hot or frigid cold. Emotional extremes appear related in part, to Pluto; whereas mental extremes are more associated with Uranus.
*Associations:* Pluto is tentatively be associated with dangerous new bacteria and the outbreak of plagues. Pluto may "rule": nuclear medicine, radiation and chemotherapy, transplants, serious poisoning (gangrene, DNA altering drugs, etc.), parasites, devouring, necrosis.
Element: Plutonium? *See Chapter 10.*

## THE NORTH LUNAR NODE: ☊

*Action:* The North Lunar Node, AKA the *Dragon's Head* gives an excess of the energy wherever posited. This node gives too much of the energy of the planet it closely conjoins. This Node's energy is: hardening, poisoning, devouring, swelling, ruthless.

*Associations*: Cancers, skin disease, leprosy, parasites, impactions, toxic build up, abscess, boils, poisons, insect and snake bites, carbuncles.Vedic astrologers implicate this node (along with Saturn and Mars) in cases of eplilepsy. Uranus might also play a part in eplilepsy due to its electrical and extreme nature. The action of this Node upon the body is quite similar to that of the planet Saturn and Pluto. See Chapter 10.

## THE SOUTH LUNAR NODE: ☋

*Action:* This Node depletes, weakens and undernourishes any planet with which is closely conjoined, or any sign it is in. *The Dragon's Tail* is draining, diminishing, suggests poor defenses, and is quite sexual.

*Associations*: Mental illness, mold, vermin, parasites, necrosis, possession, effects of being hexed, gangrene, sepsis, compulsively sexual, STDs, viruses, paranoia, drug addictions of a wasting type, wasting diseases, poisoning, insect stings, malnourishment. The action of the South Node on the body is similar to that of Neptune (weak and lax). *See Chapter 10.*

## "PARS FORTUNA", THE PART OF FORTUNE ⊗

This important *part* reflects the precise Moon phase at birth as projected from the degree of the natal Ascendant (See: *The Part of Fortune in Astrology* by Judith Hill).

"Pars" has many significations, and is an essential position in the natal chart. From a health standpoint, the conjunction of this part will act to soften or correct the condition any planet in distress. Never expect a full force pathology to occur should Pars Fortuna be closely conjunct a poorly placed planet.

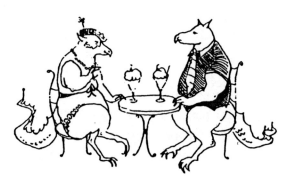

The Lunar Nodes are always opposite.

# The Houses of Health

**The First House**

The body and general constitution. According to Davidson, the ascendant sign qualifies the resistance to incoming planetary energies. Earth and Fire signs have the greatest resistance. Cancer and Pisces are the most sensitive risings to incoming force; and Air signs conduct electrical force quickly. The medical astrologer must examine this house carefully.

*The natal placement by sign and house of the planet ruling the natal ascendant sign* is essential in assessing the general state of the body. An ascendant ruler poorly placed by sign or in malefic houses 6, 8, 12, suggests that extra precaution will be necessary throughout life to maintain good health. A poorly placed ascendant ruler becomes a first choice candidate for "Upaye", the Vedic system of gem remedies (Chapter 21).

**The Sixth House - "the house of health"**

This is the house of general health interests, maintenance and support of the body, nursing. Possible weak or compromised areas of the body. Planets in this house may represent health issues.

According to the Vedic tradition, Saturn and Mars strengthen the immune system and general health when natally in this house, giving good resistance, and often excellent health. Personally, I have often found this ofttimes true, long before learning of the Vedic tradition. This does not stop these planets from producing accidents or problems due their own nature, if afflicted.

Conversely, Vedic tradition reports that Jupiter, our good guy, is not so good in this region, bringing serious illnesses. Once again, I was often puzzled by the serious illness seen in charts of clients with "benefic" Jupiter in the 6th or 8th house, only later learning the Vedic tradition!

The ruling planet of this house has much to do with health matters. Planets this ruler conjoins and/or the natal house it tenants may be colored by both health matters and health interests. For instance, the ruler of the 6th house posited in the 1st house indicates a considerable interest in health practices, but also definite health issues in life.

**The Eighth House**

The house of death, or all struggles to overcome the threat of death. This is the area of surgery, drastic measures, chronic ailments, diagnosis and psychological analysis. However it is also the house of transforming and cleansing. Rolfing, colonics, detoxification and all methods to turn oneself around are under the auspices of the 8th house. Notice that the symbol for the number "8" is also the symbol for eternity, when horizontally placed.

When Saturn transits this region, one has the option to struggle to turn oneself around or instead, get worse. The planetary ruler of this house afflicts any house it is posited in, and any planet it aspects. Planets tenanting this house at birth may reflect chronic complaints, or alternatively, gifts in: healing, surgery, psychology, research and diagnosis.

### The Twelfth House

This is the house of spiritual work and sleep. Psychological problems influencing health are sometimes indicated here. Also look here for hidden causes behind apparent health issues.

*Important*: This house governs sleep. Our current epidemic of sleep deficiency is paving the way to all kinds of health issues. Look here for the "sleep life" as well as the pleasure element of the sex life, according to the Vedic tradition. Mars or Mercury in Air or Fire signs or in Virgo reflect a tendency toward insomnia.

Planets in this house may be weakened or take on pathological qualities in reflex to the opposing sixth house. Psychological issues are more typical for planets in this house, especially if the planet is debilitated, retrograde or receiving poor aspects.

The ruler of this house may weaken or undermine any natal planet it conjoins or house it tenants. This negative effect would be offset if the ruler of the 12th house is dignified and well aspected.

Jupiter and Venus joy in this house and if well aspected assist the entire health through a peaceful state of mind and restful sleep.

## BODY ZONES BY PLANET, SIGN AND HOUSE

In astrology, as in law, we have something called "testimony". This is when a planet suggests to the reader an astrological fact by means of its position and condition in the birth chart. One testimony of disease is never enough for confident judgment. It is said that three testimonies are needed for certainty.

In our search for a collusion of testimonies in the same direction we perform an "triune assessment of bodily systems." Each body part has

associated with it three bearers of testimony:
1) a governing sign; 2), a governing planet; 3), an associated house. (This last is easy: the first sign is linked to the first house, the second sign to the second house, and so forth through all twelve houses.)

We begin the assessment of any bodily system with its' governing sign, next we study the condition of this sign's ruling planet, and lastly, this governing sign's associated house.

**We can through this triune check discover if any one bodily region receives three pathological testimonies.**

EXAMPLE: The Planetary Health Chart of a man born with congenital heart defects might demonstrate the following: Leo, sign of the heart, holds malefic Saturn. His Sun (rules Leo and also the heart) is in detriment and simultaneously afflicted by two squares. Finally, his natal 5th House (associated with the 5th sign Leo) also rules the heart. Here we find the Moon poorly placed in Capricorn (her detriment).

*Judgment:* This man demonstrates an astrological triple whammy. The sign of the heart, the planet ruling the heart and even the house of the heart are all evidencing problems! One might foresee some problem with the heart.

Below, the triune "rulers" of each body part are listed, with extra tips.

## Body Zones by Planet, Sign and House

THE HEAD, BRAIN, UPPER JAW AND EYES: Aries, Mars, the ascendant. Also check Sun and Moon for eyesight. Certain fixed stars also influence sight and the student is wise to study their influence from other sources.

THE EAR, NOSE, THROAT, NECK, LOWER JAW: Taurus, Venus rules the mouth and cheeks although she shares the lower jaw is shared with Mars. The 2nd house (as counted from ascendant as "1" counterclockwise).
*Note:* Chronic problems in this region are often reflexes from a toxic colon (opposite sign Scorpio). Always check both Taurus as well as Scorpio for chronic sore throat, nasal infection etc.

RESPIRATORY SYSTEM, NERVES, ARMS, HANDS, SPEECH: Gemini, Mercury, 3rd house (as counted from the ascendant as "1" counterclockwise). Also check the sign Cancer for lower lung. Also, malefic influence from Pisces acts to weaken the lungs.

STOMACH, BREASTS, WOMB, MUCOUS MEMBRANE: The sign Cancer, the Moon, the 4th sign (as counted from the ascendant as "1" counterclockwise). The uterus is also strongly influenced by Scorpio. Virgo becomes involved in uterine rulership during pregnancy and labor.

HEART, BACK and SPINAL CORD: Leo, the Sun, the 5th sign (as counted counterclockwise from the ascendant as "1"). Leo and Sagittarius both seem to influence the health of the spinal cord and its sheath.

INTESTINES, PANCREAS, LIVER, IMMUNE SYSTEM: Virgo; Cancer shares sign rulership of the liver with Virgo, Jupiter is the planetary ruler of the liver. For intestines and pancreas use: Virgo, Mercury and 6th sign (as counted from the ascendant as "1" counterclockwise). The spleen is in dispute: Cancer (Davidson), Virgo (others).

KIDNEYS, ALKALINE/ACID AND HORMONAL BALANCING:
For kidneys, use: Libra, Venus and 7th sign (as counted counterclockwise from ascendant as "1"). For acid/alkaline and hormonal balance check Venus/Mars and Libra/Aries polarity.

GENITAL-URINARY SYSTEM AND COLON: Generally, Scorpio, Mars and 8th sign (as counted from the ascendant as "1", counterclockwise). Females may include Venus for genitalia. Scorpio shares rulership of the uterus with Cancer. Ovaries are Venus; 16-17° Scorpio and possibly Libra. The excretion of urine is under Mars; and 28° Libra through Scorpio rule the bladder. Libra governs the kidneys. Cornell mentions the Moon as also having some relation to the bladder vs her governance of receptacles.

SCIATIC NERVE, HIPS AND THIGHS, ARTERIAL HEALTH: Sagittarius and 9th sign (as counted from ascendant as "1") for hips and thighs. Sagittarius, Jupiter and 9th sign for arterial health. Combine with a study of Leo for blood pressure check. The spinal cord and sheath, traditionally under Leo, may also hold a relationship with Sagittarius, ruler of the sciatic nerve. Jupiter is influencial over the legs in general, although also look to Aquarius for the shin and ankle.

KNEES, SKIN, GENERAL HEALTH OF BONES, TEETH, MINERAL NUTRITION: Capricorn, Saturn, 10th sign (as counted from ascendant as "1', counterclockwise). Saturn is the minerals, whereas the Moon shows success of absorption.

CIRCULATION: Saturn impedes circulation to the sign it tenants, squares or opposes. *Capillaries*: Gemini; *veins and venous circulation*: Venus, Libra and Aquarius; *arteries and arterial circulation*: Sagittarius, Jupiter.

THE ELECTRICAL SYSTEM OF THE BODY: Aquarius, Uranus, Mercury.

FEET: Pisces, 12th house (as counted from the ascendant as "1" counterclockwise). *Note*: Mercury has more governance over the extremities an also pairs of things (i.e. shoes), than the traditional ruler of Pisces, Jupiter.

LYMPHATICS: Pisces rules the lymphatic system, whereas the Moon governs the lymph. The Thoracic Duct is under the influence of the Moon ruled sign Cancer. Cornell suggests that Aquarius may share rulership of the lymphatics with Pisces. Neptune may have some effect upon the lymph.

QUALITY OF THE BLOOD: Aquarius and Pisces are prone to deficiencies of the blood. The sign Aquarius is strongly implicated in anemia. Mars governs the hemoglobin, the iron - carrying red blood corpuscles. The lymph and white fluid in the blood is governed by Pisces. The Moon rules the waters in the body.

GLANDULAR CHECK: Venus, Moon (female hormones); Mars (male), Libra-Aries and Taurus-Scorpio are the signs most associated with the sex hormones. Cancer is a sign prone to glandular imbalances. Pisces is said to hold general dominion over the ductless glands.

*Edgar Cayce matches the glands to the planets thus: Adrenals: Mercury: Pineal; Mars; Thymus: Venus; Pituitary: Jupiter; the Gonads: Saturn; Thyroid: Uranus.*

NERVOUS SYSTEM CHECK: Gemini, Sagittarius, Virgo, Mercury, Uranus, the 3rd and 9th houses (as counted from the ascendant as "1" counterclockwise). Planets in Aquarius contribute to heightened nervous sensitivity.

THE MEMORY: Cancer and the Moon govern the memory. However, it is notable that Neptune in conjunction with Mercury can produce photographic memory but absentmindedness about normal things! The 4th and 12th houses (as counted from the ascendant as "1" counterclockwise,) *continued* are houses influencing memory storage.

THE LIVER: It appears that the liver may become sluggish when natal Jupiter resides in an Earth sign (Capricorn, Virgo and Taurus), in that order. This condition is almost certain if Jupiter is retrograde, and also receiving at least one affliction by conjunction, square, opposition or quincunx aspect from Saturn (0°, 90°, 150°, 180°); and/or a conjunction with the Lunar South Node. Liver disease is an increased potential should Jupiter be in the natal 6th or 8th houses, especially if in an earth sign.

STRENGTH: Muscular strength is indicated by a strong Mars, Saturn and curiously, Venus. Very strong people often have Saturn and/or Mars in the first two houses of the horoscope. A well placed and dignified Venus encourages strength, according to the Vedic tradition. However, Venus on her own seldom produces a Hercules. We need strong bones (Saturn) and muscle (Mars). Mars below the horizon in a female sign, especially for a night birth produces excellent stamina and athletic abilities. Mars conjunct the North Node is a fine testimony of muscular prowess. Cornell sights that "strong men" are born with Saturn rising in Leo. As a verification, the strongest person I ever encountered was so born.

VIRILITY/FERTILITY: Male virility is indicated by Mars (Western) and Venus (Vedic). Virility and masculine prowess are certainly the province of Mars. The male organs are also under his beams, reflected in his symbol. However, according to the Jyotish (astrologers of India), and also Cornell, Venus rules the semen. But Venus also governs the ovaries and female eggs to some extent (with the Moon)! Women frequently conceive when transit Mars conjoins their natal Venus, providing one testimony that it is Mars that rules the sperm (or at least its inseminating powers); whereas Venus rules the eggs. But we must keep in mind that tradition insists Venus rules the sperm, despite her usual province over exclusively feminine affairs.

Female infertility is reflected by a too "dry" or "hot" Moon under stressful aspects. A dry Moon is one in Capricorn or Virgo, and/or conjunct, square or opposing Saturn. Fire signs render the Moon too hot for optimum fertility. The Moon conjunct the Dragon's Tail is another testimony of infertility. The Moon is reflective of fertility when conjunct Venus or North Node, especially so in female signs. Taurus is perhaps the best Moon sign placement for female fertility. Cornell states that Sun rules the right ovary and Moon the left, and that Venus governs the Ovum. Libra effects the ovaries and Scorpio rules the genital region of both genders.

# The Four Elements in Medical Astrology

*Fire:* Aries, Leo, Sagittarius (masculine)
*Earth:* Taurus, Virgo, Capricorn (feminine)
*Air:* Gemini, Libra, Aquarius (masculine)
*Water:* Cancer, Scorpio, Pisces (feminine)

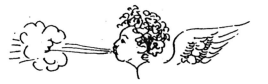

The four elements of antiquity can be seen as a structural thread running through theoretical realms as diverse as physiognomy and Jungian psychology. However, it is in Western medical astrology that the four elements stand alone in purest form, unencumbered by abstractions and theories imposed by the less physically oriented sciences. To acquaint the reader with these four elements and their use in early western medicine is the purpose of this article. First, we must introduce a few basics.

The four elements represent four planes of matter (and much more as will be described later). Classical astrology assigns each of the twelve zodiacal signs to one of the four elements: *Fire, Earth, Air, or Water.* The fiery, airy, watery, and earthy signs form our first and simplest description of zodiacal types useful to the early physicians.

At birth, the weight of planetary distribution within each of the elements paints an astrophysical portrait of the elemental balance within both psyche and body. An observation of the planetary birth map allows us to discover the weakest elements in our physical and psychological makeup and also the most dominant. Frequently, we emotionally feel and physically see the dominant element of a friend before perhaps guessing their more particular zodiac sign type.

However, what exactly are these four elements? In fact, the four elements can be viewed esoterically, spiritually, psychologically, and physically. Fire, Earth, Air and Water describe four levels of concretization of matter, four states of awareness, four temperaments and four types of matter within the chemical-molecular universe. This explains why the astrologers, Jungian psychologists, and medieval physicians, have each defined the four elements variously and utilized their knowledge of them for quite separate purposes.

*The Elements as Levels of the Concretization of Matter*
In the most arcane sense, the elements refer to four levels of

increasing concretization of matter: *photon, particle, atom and molecule.* One can think of this concretization process as the journey of light (the photon, as the Fire element) from complete freedom (Fire) into gradually denser and more predictable forms, represented first by Air and then Water; until it finds itself "trapped" in the densest plane of the molecule, symbolized as the stodgy, reliable Earth element. As the photon journeys from creation towards material expression ( particle, atom molecule), it gathers weight, experience and form while sacrificing the playfulness and freedom of the photon and particle.

*The Four Elements and the Four Worlds*

The four levels of concretization of matter directly correspond to the Four planes, or worlds of the Kabbalists. Their highest or Spiritual World , *Atziluth* is the world of emanations and archetypes. Atziluth corresponds best with the photon and with the Fire element. The second plane, *Briah*, constitutes the world of thought and creation. Briah belongs to the world of particles and to the thinking element Air. Similarly, the malleable Astral World, known to Kabbalists as *Yetzirah*, the world of formations, corresponds to the atom and the receptive, impressionable and feeling oriented Water element. Last, the Physical Plane (or Chemical-Molecular Plane) is the realm of the molecule and is represented by the densest element Earth. Kabbalists know this fourth world as *Assiah*, the world of action and the world of matter. As denizens of Assiah, we find ourselves at present confined largely to the laws of the material plane.

*The Four Elements as Four Types of Consciousness*

The four elements are also commonly described as four types of consciousness. Jung, who studied astrology and read horoscopes, adopted these traditional four awareness as his famous four psychological types. However, these four types are neither Jung's invention, or anything new to astrologers whom have used them for millennia.

*Fire* symbolizes pure being, the sense of "I", and the life force. It is direct experience. Jung made this his famous "intuitive" type.

*Air* represents the intellect. This is the world of thought, language and abstraction. Its mode of consciousness is detached observation. Jung renamed Air his "thinking" type.

Our receptive feeling function is *Water*. Emotions and instincts arise from this level. Water is responsive and subjective experience. A person with this form of type of awareness Jung termed a "feeling" type.

*Earth* represents sensation, and the body. This is the densest of the four levels and corresponds to body consciousness, materiality, survival and the structuring body building function. Jung christened Earth as his "Sensate" type.

### The Four Temperaments

Medieval physicians classified four humors of the body, and associated these with four physiognomical and temperamental types termed Choleric (Fire), Sanguine (Air), Phlegmatic (Water) and Melancholic (Earth). We do not have the space here to commence a detailed discussion of these four humors and corresponding temperaments.

It is enough to say that the four temperaments although also physiognomical, do roughly correspond to "Jung's" four astrologically based psychological types, although in some writings the Melancholic or Earth type is viewed as entirely negative, which is inaccurate.

In this system, a balance of the four humors produced a balanced temperament and a state of good health. Disease was a manifestation of an imbalance of these humors. A similar idea continues today in modern Ayurvdic practice, with one exception. The four humors of the body have been grouped into just three "doshas". Air becomes *Vata*, Fire is *Pitta*, and Water and Earth combine in a single "heavy" humor known as *Kapha*. The description of the Kapha type appears to combine the qualities of both the traditional western Phlegmatic and Melancholic psychological temperaments.

Fruits, vegetables, medicines and activities are also classed under each dosha. Healing is assisted by subscribing to a regimen that balances these doshas, or elemental forces. If you are too hot, then you must cool off. If you are too damp, then you must dry out, and so forth.

### The Four Elements as Four Types of Matter

This is very simple. The element Fire manifests as fire. The element Air as air. Water is water, and Earth is literally earth. However their correspondences to the physical body are a bit more complex.

*Fire* is the Chinese "Chi" or vital force, also the energy and the digestive force. Fire releases energy. Therefore,the metabolic and fuel burning activities of the body take place through activation of the Fire element. The action of Fire is hot, light and dry.

*Air* governs the little known electrical forces and electrical connections within the body, neurotransmission, motion, oxygenation of the blood, breath, language and motion. Its action is cold, light and moist

(some texts say alternatively cold, light and dry.)

*Water* rules the waters of the body, including the phlegm, the lymph, semen, blood and all bodily secretions and fluids. The moist and protective mucous membranes of the body are a function of the Water element. Also, our memory function is related to Water because Water is the most impressionable of elements. The action of Water upon the body is cold heavy and wet.

*Earth* governs the minerals within the body, the bones and the building up of a bodily structure. Earth also holds in energy, and has much to do with stamina, food storage, body building, and longevity. Earth is warm, heavy and dry (the Earth sign Taurus may be an exception, producing more a warm and moist condition.) Natives of Taurus, the preeminent Earth sign are noted for being human greenhouses, always maintaining a warm body temperature.

THE FOUR ELEMENTS: A SUMMARY

To reiterate, the four elements are *four states or qualities of matter*: that of light, liquid, gaseous, and solid. As said earlier, each of the twelve signs are assigned to one of the four elements. This classification is accomplished in the following manner: *Fire:* Aries, Leo, Sagittarius; *Air:* Gemini, Libra, Aquarius; *Water:* Cancer, Scorpio, Pisces; *Earth:* Taurus, Virgo, Capricorn.

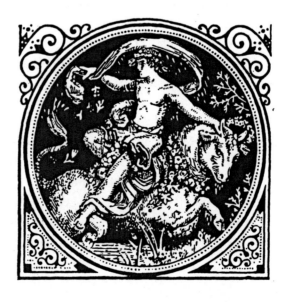

# Imbalances of the Four Elements and Health

Imbalance of the four elements occurs in one of two ways: *deficiency or excess*. Your planetary birth chart is the tool used by astrologers to divine the quality and amount of each element in the birth chart. Until the mid-17th century, physicians were required to have passed their exams in astrology. Each physician was expected to be fluent in the diagnosis of planetary charts from the medical perspective.

Included here is a listing of common complaints associated with both the excesses and deficiencies of each element. A few interesting cases from my own files will round out the discussion.

FIRE: *Excess*
Dehydration, hyperactivity, hyperthyroid, baldness.
emaciation, great hunger, brainstorms, aneurism, heart attack, high blood pressure, stroke, overheating, sunstroke, insomnia, liver disturbances, ego mania, compulsive behaviors, itch, inflammation, alcoholism, boils, acne eruptions, arterial and blood vessel complaints, hyper stress.

*Antidote for Fire Excess*: The Water element.
*Treatments*: Hydration with cool liquids, cool baths, cool moist herbs and foods, sweet and moist foods, fruits, green color, calm music, avoid hot spicy and oily foods, avoid red colors, stay away from hot sun, avoid overheating, apply liver tonics and purification, strengthen arteries, avoid temper and excessive excitement.

FIRE: *Deficiency*
Weak, listless, overweight, low blood pressure, depression, poor eyesight, poor self esteem, fatigued, poor digestive fire, weak heart.

*Balance for Fire Deficiency*: Apply Fire, Earth, Air.
*Treatments*: Exercise, heart and blood tonics, red stones and colors, dance and play therapy, brass instruments and rousing music, iron, spices, improve circulation, develop muscles of upper body, sing, paint. Increase oxygen. Pranayama. Mineral therapies. Increase protein, iron, minerals.

*Field Notes: Fire*
Here is an interesting case of Fire *excess* extracted from the files.

A friend of mine gave birth to a redheaded baby boy. Soon after birth he became badly dehydrated, fitful and would rage all night. He had great difficulty sleeping.

His birth chart showed not only an excess of the astrological hot and dry Fire signs but none of the balancing moist Water signs, plus also a very prominent Mars near the ascendant at birth. (Mars of course, is a hot and dry planet). Upon hearing this, the mother had the invention and insight to do something to bring the Water element into the baby's energy field. She began soaking him in a comfortable bath just before bed! Baby loved his baths and afterward slept sweetly, his crying problem greatly diminished from the onset of the water "experiments".

Fire *deficiency* frequently manifests as a lack of confidence and a weak ego. The individual lacks playfulness, warmth, creativity and pizzazz. One may also lack the ability to initiate activities. One case of *deficient* Fire combined with excess Earth is most interesting. This man suffered from an absolutely compulsive need to seek stimulating entertainment and social events. It was as if he craved stimulation (Fire) from outside because he could not find it within. However, despite his constant socializing, he was personally so introverted and reserved that he could hardly carry on a conversation and had the greatest difficulty expressing himself in any way, or displaying affection.

Outwardly, he appeared cold, rather lifeless and unresponsive. Inwardly he possessed much stamina (Earth), and was a capable long distance runner.

AIR: *Excess*
Scattered, nervous, excess talking, mentally unbalanced
or fatigued, mental flights, hyperactive, restless, cold, anemia arthritic, hypersensitive, emaciated, unstable, thin and balding hair, lacks personality force, weakness, self destructive through irregular living, indecisive, scattered.

*Antidote for Excess Air:* Earth
*Treatments*: Good nutrition, Mineral baths and tonics, warmth, nature, massage, practicality, gain weight, business training, weight lifting, warm solid and well prepared meals a day, warm grains, root foods, calming music, quiet time, sleep, sedatives, nervousness and mental rest, yellow and blue colors.

AIR: *Deficiency*

Asthma, sub oxygenation of cells, lung weakness, poor judgment, lack of humor, listless, overly intense (Air lightens), slow in thought or movement, poor circulation, weak heart action, low blood pressure.

*Balance for Air Deficiency:* Air, Fire. Breathing exercises, improve bodily oxygenation and circulation, humor therapy, views, mental development exercises, fresh air, juggling, coordination exercises, speech therapy, flexibility exercises, yoga, strengthen the lungs and arms, build strength.

*Field Notes: Air*

Over the years a number of clients have arrived with *deficient* Air element. I always then ask the question "Do you have asthma, shortness of breath or bronchitis?" Their reply is typically affirmative. It is evident that Air deficient people do indeed lack oxygen!

Lack of Air may also manifest on the mental plane as a lack of levity, comparative reasoning or objectivity. A recent case was that of a young woman with many talents. However, she could not acquire appropriate schooling for lack of ability with tests and memorization of facts. She simply could not learn through the standard western educational method. She took readily to my suggestion that she might do better in an experimental type of educational setting.

Air *excess* produces the scattered, unsettled and over talkative individual. This type does spurns routine and does not take care good of themselves. Smoking cigarettes, irregular sleeping, sexual and eating habits, plus frequent job changes all give rise to fatigued nerves and an unsettled mental condition. Although seemingly able to burn the candles at both ends without mishap, the Air type will burn themselves out early and not infrequently expires before their time.

Tuberculosis, nervous breakdown, mental disturbances and malnutrition are complaints common to excess Air especially when coupled with a deficient Earth element. In cases of excess Air, the Ayurvedic physicians insists on a stable routine combined with warm grains, oils and vegetables. Cold foods and beverages are verboten as are excess and excesses of all kinds.

WATER: *Excess*

Water retention, bloat, nausea, fermentations, yeast, sluggishness, low energy, oversleeping, drowsy, over sexed, indulgent, dependent and addictive behaviors, obese, paranoid, tender swellings, pain sensitive, overly emotional and childish, lazy, depressed, chills, weak eyesight, poor structure and posture, weak teeth and bones, shuns daylight, avoids reality, introversion, noise sensitivity, soft growths and tumors, breast lumps, prostrate swellings, excess mucous and other bodily fluids, avoids reality.

*Antidote for Water Excess*: Fire
*Treatments:* Purgatives, sweats, promote urination, hot spices, exercise, dry heat, heat lamps, cognitive therapy, sunlight, laughter, warm colors,stimulation, affection. Avoid cold wet and sweet foods (ice cream and watermelon are the worst for this type), improve heart action and circulation. The Water type responds excellently to kindness.

WATER: *Deficiency*:

Insomnia, restless and overactive, dehydrated, dry, inability to relax, constipated, infertile, low libido or sex satisfaction, fears or alternatively craves intimacy, low appetites, insensitive, memory dysfunction, paranoia, complaints of dryness, swallowing, etc.

*Balance for Water Deficiency*: Apply Water.
*Treatments:* Swim and bathe, humidifiers, drink liquids,exposure to Moonlight, pearls, silver, dolphins, puddings and custards, romantic music, sleep, sedatives, psychotherapy, psyllium seed, slippery elm bark, chanting, herbal laxatives, comfrey root and similar demulcents to moisten the mucous membranes, aphrodisiacs, nurturing (receiving or giving), support groups, lakes, rivers and oceans, boating, fishing, meditating, devotional and charitable work.

*Field Notes: Water*

In my work a number of interesting cases have appeared of persons born with a great excess in the Water signs. In most of these cases, should a lack of the drying Fire element also fail to be present, you will find the dropsical and water laden body.

Two cases demonstrate *Water excess* most effectively. One case was of a girl who spent most of her life in a semi coma following a botched operation for brain tumor. This unfortunate individual was very sensitive, sweet and passive, and eventually passed on at a young age. A similar case of being "under water" is that of Helen Keller, born deaf, dumb and blind. She was also born with a considerable excess of planets in the astrological

Water signs. However, despite her unusual condition this individual achieved much and the malady appeared to be restricted to the physical condition.

Three cases of Water deficiency recently observed produced individuals who suffered from a lack of *inner peace*. Water is the element of peace, and so this makes good sense. Both individuals were restless, suffered insomnia and found it impossible to relax or to enjoy intimacy.

One friend who completely lacked the Water element and yet possessed much Fire, compulsively spent her money and traveled. This strange behavior was symptomatic of too much throwing off type energy (Fire, Air), and not enough holding in type energy (Earth, Water). She was seized with intense ambitions that would abruptly change with the wind. Her dry and hard body completely lacked the subcutaneous fat typical of the feminine sex. In this case, a medieval physician might attempt to introduce the Water and possibly Earth elements into the body while simultaneously cooling down the Fire element, and balancing the Air element.

Earth: *Excess*

Mental dullness, lack of mental creativity, either boring or suffers a chronic sense of boredom, withholding, laconic, overeats and overworks, the body is either sluggish and very large and heavy or very bony and emaciated (curious! The weight extreme observed will depend on a number of other factors). Suffers dryness, constipation, dandruff, skin problems, excema, brittle nails and cuticles (dry), mucous membranes also dry, brittle teeth, hearing problems. Unresponsive and insensitive. Generally strong and healthy on a daily level, although highly prone to chronic conditions and cancer due to toxic buildups, constipation, arthritis and rheumatism, bone spurs, hard growths, cancer. Great longevity.

*Antidote for Earth Excess*: Fire, Air then Water.
*Treatments:* Purgatives, colonic therapy, fasting, vegetarianism, saunas, emotional and affectional development, light eating of light foods, flexibility exercises, dexterity exercises, oil rubs and compresses, conversation, variety, travel, mental stimulation (improve mental speed, verbal and comparative faculties), humor, neurological stimulation, development of social fluidity, demulcent herbs to moisten the mucous membranes, *avoidance* of rich, toxic or dry foods such as meat, milk products and pastries, breathing exercises, views and flying, reading and writing, hatha yoga.

Earth: *Deficiency*

Difficulty in gaining or holding weight or money, low stamina, weak bones and teeth, poor physical strength and endurance, weak posture and bodily structure, poor appetite, nervous, impractical, unstable, cold, insufficient immunity, hypothermia, cold body, malnutrition, mineral deficiency, ungrounded.

*Balance for Earth Deficiency*: Apply Earth

*Treatments:* Minerals, mud and mineral baths, nature, sitting on the Earth, hatha yoga, stable routine, weight lifting, aikido, Tai Chi and other exercises that teach one to hold in energy, warmth, massage and touch, steady jobs, herbal therapies, calcium, good food, gardening, building, pottery, sculpture, business training and money management, improve attention to clothing and appearance.

*Field Notes: Earth*

As in other elements, an excess or deficiency of Earth becomes more apparent with the simultaneous appearance of an opposite condition for another element.

Two individuals that spring to mind possessing excess Earth and low Fire are very simple and uncomplex personalities, slow moving and yet thorough and dedicated in all endeavors undertaken. Their bodies are also dense and sluggish, as is their speech. One of the two suffered a hearing complaint, typical of Earth signs. Their bones, hands and feet were large, and clumsy. Physically, they were always very warm. Remember, the Earth is a greenhouse, it holds in heat, whereas Fire lets it out! Earth is a very tough, dense element and so are excessively Earthy people.

It is not therefore unremarkable that a number of the great heavy weight boxers (including Rocky Marciano, Foreman, Frasier and Muhammad Ali) were born in Earth signs. It would be interesting to make a statistical study of Earth signs in the birth charts of boxers. Curiously, other Earth type people I've observed are of the bony "ectomorphic" category. This is due to the rulership of Saturn over the Earth sign Capricorn. This Saturnian type Earth element person may be bony but they are dependably tough and strong, with excellent stamina.

A case of Earth *deficiency* with strong Air came with a man who was finding it impossible to find a home. And although he made good money, *stability* evaded him. Neither did he understand money or the material universe very well and was ever in danger of being conned by the more worldly wise. Mentally he was agitated and fearful of dealing with life's realities. Remember, Earth signs deal with the earth plane! Sometimes he would forget to eat, and possessed no materialistic desire to own anything.

His body was exceptionally fragile, and he suffered a lifelong trouble with stamina (Earth element), rendering him incapable of prolonged physical labor. He could do anything a little while, but just could not physically keep up on the long hike. It was important to him to spend time in nature (Earth) everyday. Nature calmed his sensitive nerves and provided the quiet he longed for more than anything else.

He tended to insufficient digestion of nutrients leading to mineral deficiencies and benefited from minerals taken through sea water extracts. Earthy staples such as grains and potatoes were favorite foods although he could not eat too much at one sitting without difficulty. It was important for him to lift weights only to maintain his delicate frame in good health. Curiously, he was greatly attracted to granite and other heavy rocks and loved to sit on boulders overlooking natural scenes.

As a rule, he suffered greatly from cold and seemed unable to produce or contain his own heat. Hypothermia was ever a danger. The only way he could warm up was through application of hot baths and a glass of hot tea before bed. In all probability, a medieval physician would have him apply hot earth, mud or mineral compresses to replenish the missing Earth element.

*The Elements in Combination*

The above descriptions are uncomplex compared to the actual practice of medical astrology. The four elements are never observed in a vacuum. Any elemental excess present in the planetary birth chart automatically signals the reader that some other element must be deficient. This fact gives rise to several classifications of deficient/excess element pairs, too numerous to discuss in this present article.

Additionally, the entire birth chart is taken under consideration. The planets in particular are observed for sign placement, and also according to their temperature, hearkening back to, and supportive of the four elements. For instance, Mars is a hot and dry planet and Saturn is cold and dry. However, should you be born at night, with Mars appearing above the horizon and in a cooling Water or Earth sign, then the normally destructive nature of Mars is toned down through his cooler, moister situation. Similarly, Saturn benefits by placement in a warming day birth, especially when placed above the horizon in a warm masculine sign.

*Field Notes: A Case of Elements Acting Together*

An extremely interesting case recently came to my attention.

This is the case of a young man with an excess of both Earth and Fire, acting in combination with a condition which can only be described as *disturbed* Water.

The disturbed Water element was brought about in the following manner: the moist Moon was in the hot and dry Fire element, and strongly afflicted by Mars, a hot, drying planet. To compound matters, Mars was the only planet located in the Water element. This created an extremely dry and agitated condition within the body.

Repeatedly, the boy was hospitalized for severe dehydration. He could not drink or eat and his stomach rejected not only foods but liquids. Severe constipation, difficulty swallowing and partial deafness accompanied the foregoing symptoms. Remember, Water rules the mucous membranes, and in this boy's case Water was not only weak but suffers from an *intrusion* of the Fire element, further damaging Water's soothing and moisturizing properties.

The excess of Earth in the birth chart created a dry, dull and listless appearance.

The Air element was also weak, exacerbating the combination of excess Earth and Fire with disturbed Water. As a rarified element, Air acts to assist the burning rate of Fire, which otherwise smolders intensely without enough Air. Also, a satisfactory Air element would prevent the Earth element from becoming too heavy and absorbing. Could the ancient elemental medicine bring relief for this unfortunate case?

*Conclusion*

The medical use of the ancient four elements continues to the present time in two forms. In the East, the respected practice of Ayurvedic medicine heavily relies upon the consideration of the doshas (elements) for diagnosis and treatment. In Europe, the entirety of medical astrology inclusive of the four medical elements was forced underground at the close of the 17th century. However, despite the prevailing opposition against the practice of Western astro-medicine, it is utilized by a small number of licensed Western physicians.

Davidson's excellent medical *Lectures*, (out of print) and Cornell's (Dr.) *Encyclopedia of Medical Astrology* are but a few cases in point. One cannot peruse the contents of these writings without being suitably impressed with the complexity and sophistication of 20th century medical astrology.  Other interesting examples might be Dr. Millard's *Case notes of a Medical Astrologer,* and Carl Jansky's *Modern Medical Astrology.*

Those that practice medical astrology are certain of its efficacy. Personally, I've witnessed cases where the cause of a hidden health complaint eludes the doctors while the answer sits crystal clear in the horoscope  waiting to be seen by all. Eventually, and after many tests, if not enormous cost to the hapless patient, the doctors finally discover the source of the mystery problem to be identical with the astrologer's diagnosis. Could it be that the ancient physicians were on to something after all?

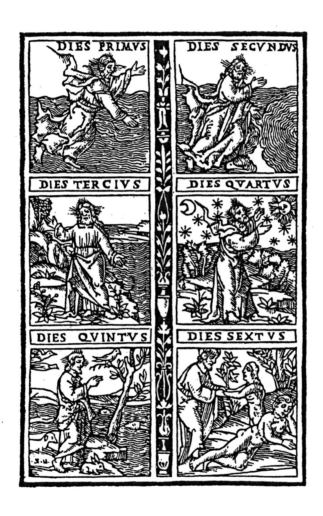

# The Astrological Modes: The Rate of Matter in Motion and the Flow of the Vital Force.

There is a further sign classification of great import. We already know that the four elements represent four types of matter and also four kinds of energy. Because matter moves, we must sub-designate each element (type of matter) according to the *rate of matter in motion*. This subdivision produces the three *modes*, also known as the *quadruplicities* of classical Western astrology. It is these three modes that describe the *rate of matter in motion*.

These three rates of motion are known as the *Cardinal, Mutable and Fixed modes*. Simply put, these rates are: fast, low and meandering.

For instance, Fire igniting is *Cardinal Fire*, whereas the concentrated fire of an oven becomes *Fixed Fire* in action. A wild fire would be similar in nature to *Mutable Fire*, or moving fire.

*Cardinal* energy is *fast*. Signs of the *Cardinal* mode exist as a pure expression of their element and always lead the season. The equinoxes and solstices occur at the onset of a Cardinal sign. *Fixed* energy is *slow*, always occurs in mid-season, when energy is most concentrated. *Mutable* energy is *fluctuating and dispersive*, always occurring at the end of a season as it gradually changes into the following quarter.

So we now see that any one of these four elements, (or types of vital force) can move in one of three ways, or modes.

## Nature of the Three Modes

**The Cardinal Mode** or *quadruplicity:* Aries, Cancer, Libra, Capricorn. *Cardinal* signs always begin the season and bring *decisive shifts of energy*. These signs are activating. (One may well argue the reverse is true in the case of indecisive Libra or introverted Cancer if one fails to observe that Libra *initiates* the Air qualities of abstract contemplativeness and detached observation; whereas Cancer activates feeling and responsiveness, the very essence of the Water element).

Cardinal signs begin action. *The Cardinal Mode suggests acute conditions.*

**The Fixed Mode** or *quadruplicity:* Taurus, Leo, Scorpio, Aquarius.

The *Fixed* signs are the stubborn four because these signs concentrate that season's elemental energy. Their energy is slow, enduring and hard to change like an old oak tree. Fixed signs always occur midseason when that season's energy is most concentrated. *Chronic conditions are indicated.*

**Mutable Mode** or *quadruplicity:* Gemini, Virgo, Sagittarius, Pisces.

*Mutable* signs are noted for their versatile, flexible and sometimes unstable natures.

Mutable signs always occur at the transition point between two seasons and are therefore fluctuating and meandering in nature. The Mutable mode disperses and translates energy. Mutable signs, particularly Pisces and Gemini, seem forever in the process of morphing into something else. These signs are fluctuating and flexible like willow trees, undulating in nature. *Mutable brings the wasting, lingering and nervous ailments.*

**Mode: Qualification of Health Condition**

The mode indicates the rate of flow for the astrological element. The element describes a type of matter. To repeat, the mode then defines the rate of motion for that particular type of matter defined by an element (Fire, Air, Earth or Water), but also the flow of that life force (fast, slow, or fluctuating)

A great emphasis in any one mode might predispose one to conditions of any one of the signs of that quadruplicity.

 A Cardinal emphasis indicates acute, inflammatory conditions.

 A Fixed dominance denotes chronicity.

Mutable charts tend toward lingering, wasting and fluctuating illness.

For students of Ayurvedic medicine, the western modes closely relate to the three "doshas": Cardinal being *rajas*; Fixed, *tamas*; and Mutable, *satwa*. The fastest acting and resolved diseases are *Cardinal*.

**Rule: The mode of the Sun combined with the house position of the Sun describes on the quantity and quality of the vital force.**

Sol, our Sun is the foremost giver of life. He the center of our solar system and likewise, the center of your birth chart. The condition of Sol in the birth chart tells us of the quality and quantity of natural Vital Force, or "chi" we were born with. Some signs have more chi than others. The martial signs Aries and Scorpio possess much chi force. Taurus the Bull is allotted the greatest contained magnetic force, and longevity of all signs.

The burn rate of the vitality varies greatly between signs, being fastest in Fire signs (Aries, Leo, Sagittarius), and slowest in Earth signs (Taurus especially, followed by Capicorn and then Virgo.)

It is thought that we are each given a set amount of vital force at birth and we burn this force at different rates. Some of us are fast burn, others, slow and steady. There are many types of "chi", the vital force. Our Sun's position by sign, house and geometric relationship with other planets tells us something about the amount and quality of our natural life force.

## MUTABLE SUN SIGNS AND CADENT HOUSES

**The *Mutable* signs: Gemini, Virgo, Sagittarius, Pisces.**
Traditionally, the Sun in a Mutable sign and also in a *cadent* astrological house (below) gives a weaker life force. In such a condition, the whole system is more delicate and prone to sensitivity, especially the immune system, nerves and lungs. "Double Mutable", as described here, is prone to lingering conditions and gradual wasting diseases. Such individuals need to observe vigilance when ill and acquire extra chi from herbs, breathing exercises, reiki or whatever works.
**Your Sun is *cadent* if located in the birth chart's 12th, 3rd, 6th or 9th sign from the ascendant** (counting the Ascendant sign as "1" and moving counterclockwise.) But to qualify as "double Mutable" Sol must also be in the Mutable signs!

## FIXED SUN SIGNS IN ANGULAR or SUCCEDENT HOUSES

**The *Fixed* family of signs: Taurus, Leo, Scorpio and Aquarius** are enhanced near the angles and when in succedent houses.

A Fixed mode Sun, in an *angular* or *succedent* directional position gives great stamina, strength, endurance plus a slow - burning life force. Longevity is common but unfortunately, so is chronic and/or life threatening illness. (Because the life force is so strong and stable, there is a greater tendency to collect and hold the toxins).
***Angular* positions are: the ascendant sign, the 4th, 7th and 10th signs as counted from the ascendant sign as "1", counterclockwise.**
***Special note:* The latter sign, Aquarius, has by far, the weakest vital force of the four Fixed signs and could be discounted if in a cadent house (see preceding paragraph) or the 4th or 7th angle. The vital force of Aquarius seems in many cases transferred from the body to the mind!**

A Fixed Sunlocated in *succedent* houses has exceptional strength of the slow burning order. **The *succedent* positions in the chart are** the 2nd, 5th, 8th and 11th signs as counted from the Ascendant as "1", moving counterclockwise.

Trust a Fixed Sun in the 8th house as having the force of will and energy to overcome even the most life threatening ailments! Scorpio is the best sign for achieving victory over death. Scorpio energy excels over all other signs as a transforming force.

## CARDINAL SUN SIGNS AND CARDINAL OR FIXED HOUSES

The *Cardinal* family of signs: **Aries, Cancer, Libra and Capricorn** are enhanced near or on the *angles* (the Ascendant, and the 4th, 7th and 10th signs as counted from the ascendant counterclockwise).

An Aries Sun possesses the greatest outward moving vital force, the more so when angular, the 7th angle being weakest. Cancer is by far, the lowest in vitality of this group. A birth Sun placed in a Cardinal sign near an angle provides a fast sparking energy, but not the sustain shown in the Fixed signs. The Cardinal sign Capricorn is the great exception, providing the slow burn and endurance usually noted for Fixed signs. However, Capricorn rarely shows this strength in youth as do Fixed signs, but in the mature years. Libra is a curiosity, in appearing outwardly unambitious and relaxed. The Cardinality of Libra is demonstrated in vivid sociality.

Cardinal Suns in succedent houses are dependably strong and give good vital force, with the exception of the Sun in Libra or Cancer in the 8th house.

### OTHER COMBINATIONS OF THE SUN'S MODE AND HOUSE

Not all combinations of the natal Sun's quadruplicity and house position are listed here. Mention is made only of combinations that produce extreme results of one type or another, as indicated.

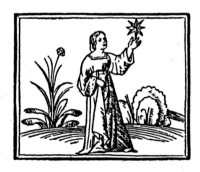

# Transits and Progressions: The Assessment of Time

From the standpoint of health, the astrological birth chart can be seen as a garden with seeds lying dormant in the ground. Only when the appropriate season arrives do the seeds sprout and produce either weeds or roses as the case may be. Of course, this is a metaphor for poor health or good health. More importantly, negative planetary weather would do less harm if we have taken precautions to prevent the seeds of ill health from sprouting in the first place!

A birth chart may possess any number of *signatures*, i.e. planetary configurations typical for various health conditions. And yet the native may appear in robust health until one fine day a wave of ideal "planetary weather" sprouts the dormant seeds of the disease potential. The resultant disease would be a near certainty if the individual had also spent their years breaking the laws of health. Conversely, someone who has taken good care of their bodily vehicle may not experience the extremity of disease of their more careless comrades.

Let us pretend there are identical twins whose birth charts demonstrate a strong astrological signature for diabetes. One child is reared on junk food and allowed to become obese. He appears healthy enough until the age of 35 when the planets "trigger" the signature by presenting the perfect astrological conditions necessary for the pancreas to malfunction. The dormant potential of diabetes now hatches into the full sail symptoms of disease.

Twin number two is raised on a healthy diet with few sweets and maintains a normal weight. The astrologically savvy parents, aware of the diabetic tendency, reinforce his pancreas with the proper herbs. In this case, the planets may never act to trigger the diabetic signature unless it is a very extreme signature indeed.

There are many variants to this scenario. Some charts seem to allow more slack, while other horoscopes demonstrate physical conditions that appear quite fixed, as if the hand of an immutable karma was at work.

There is a gulf between possessing an innate tendency toward diabetes and being born with a club foot!

## Progressions Versus Transits

Astrological *progressions* are internal timing devices. The birth positions of your planets are *progressed* forward at various rates (there are many methods). Think about the acorn of an oak tree. This seed contains not only genetic material, but timing. The first acorns, the tree's life span and various other junctures and seasons for the tree are pre-programmed in the tiny acorn.

The birth chart is representative of the human acorn! The progressions, when "due", i.e. creating exact aspects to the planets in your radix; or perhaps *ingressing* (moving into new signs) signal the astrologer that an *internal readiness* is at hand.

Rarely, do progressed aspects bring about a health change on their own. They require a "trigger" from current planetary conditions. These current planetary conditions are called *transits*. Transits often bring to a progression to fruition early or late, by up to as much as one year in either direction. The internal readiness as shown by the progression normally waits for the *transit* to bring the *external* conditions necessary for the change to occur on the physical level. One might "feel" the progressions inwardly but witness no external result until the transit planets agree.

The two most widely used progressed techniques are known as *secondary directions,* and *solar arc.* Secondary directions, i.e. a day for a year of life, is a powerful technique. It is recommended that you limit your use of progressions to one or both of these methods. It is all you will need for this study. *I might add that one can do very fine medical astrology without the use of progressions because transits are the main thing. However, if you want to perfect yourself in this study, learn to include at the Secondary Progressions and also the Solar Arc. Progression add weight to the testimony of transit timing and assist you in establishing severity.*

When a transiting planet and a progressed planet sit over the same weak link in the birth chart, you can be reasonably sure that "something" is cooking. The health sensitivity suggested by the weak link is no longer dormant and may hatch. Not only is the native internally ready for the issue or event, but the transit is now adding the weight of the current planetary weather.

It is not the place of this book to teach the reader how to calculate progressions or to use the transits. This section is for the intermediate and advanced student who has acquired this knowledge from other sources. A good beginner text for Secondary Progressions is Llewelleyn George's classic *The A to Z Horoscope Maker and Delineator.*

It is worth reiterating that you can do a perfectly accurate medical astrology diagnoses without the use of progressions. However, try not to allow ignorance of or discomfort with progressions to discourage you from studying or practicing this art.

## AN EXAMPLE OF USING TRANSITS AND PROGRESSIONS TOGETHER TO TIME ONSET, page 100.

This is a hypothetical chart I've calculated to demonstrate how transits act to trigger a progressed aspect made to a natal planet.

**Step one:** Study the Planetary Health Chart and be aware of any unusual emphasis within bodily systems or regions. Note the inherent weaknesses. You should know the sign positions of Saturn, Mars and the South Node. Be aware of the element, mode or any other unique emphasis. Make an assessment the bodily systems, as has been given in Chapter 13.

Our example chart demonstrates a great weight of planets in Aries and Taurus, the signs of the head, ears, teeth and neck. Because of the time of birth, this chart is so laid out to also emphasize the 1st and 2nd houses, which also related to these same bodily regions. We will be noting this regional emphasis and watching for a progression that might signal "now!" for onset of issues in one of these body parts.

**Step two:** Note if there are any current on near upcoming progressions to a possible health indication in the birth chart.
*Note:* If progressions scare you, then skip to Step three, the transits. Transits will work without progressions but not vice versa!

Our example chart shows us that in July of the 7th year of this child's life, we note that the Sun, (the most important of all progressed positions), moves to precisely conjoin the natal position of Saturn at 19° Taurus in the second house. I've noted this progression on the outside of the natal circle in a box, dated.

**Step three:** You will need an ephemeris for the year in which the progression is due, or (if you are not using progressions) the period of observation. Transits are watched for the transit movement of any planet from Mars outward; or any eclipse, to the degree of Saturn (in our sample chart). Use only the "hard" aspects of: conjunction (0°), square (90°) or opposition (180°).

Any natal planet in a health - sensitive condition may become your focus. In our sample chart we are focusing on Saturn, only because this is where the emphasis now is, and because Saturn is always fundamental.

*The above formulae you will always use for finding any progression's "trigger dates" as triggered by the transiting planet(s).* Transiting planets must pass over at least one of these above points to trigger the progression. To reiterate, the triggering planet must conjunct, square or oppose the degree of the progressed natal hard aspect. ("Soft" aspects i.e. the sextile (60°) or trine (120°) may not be depended upon as to trigger progressions.)

We turn our ephemeris to July, 2007. Now we scan the months on either side of July 2007, looking for sixth months on either side, and searching for the nearest month to our "due date" of July 2007, that produces a powerful transit by hard aspect to the Sun's progression of the Natal Saturn at 19° of Taurus. Again, your strongest triggers are: transit Mars, eclipses, transit Sun, transit Jupiter, Saturn or outer planets.

We find that on May 10th, the transit Sun crosses 19° Taurus by conjunction exactly as transiting Saturn achieves 18° of Leo, thus forming a perfect hard square aspect to the natal Saturn in Taurus.

Transit Saturn, (a transit of preeminent importance) moves to 19° Leo between May 20th and June 4th of the same year. (It is worth your while to always consider the degree *after* your trigger degree of equal importance. Think of a car passing a truck on the highway - you feel the breeze just after pulling out.) We can therefore extend the transit of Saturn through the 20th degree - which takes us through June 17th. The transits are drawn on the outer wheel, dated.

However, the transit triggers keep coming! Mars, our grand trigger, achieves his transit by conjunction of 19° Taurus (one degree on either side) between the dates of July 21 and 24. The conjunction is the strongest aspect of all. By July, 2007, we find a Transit Mars conjoins a Progressed Sun, and both are conjunct the Natal Saturn in Taurus, in the second house.

SO WHAT HAPPENED?

How might the above date sequence work out? This is a hypothetical scenario, typical of many observed by the author.

A child is born with a tendency for teeth problems, as shown by Saturn in the sign and house of the teeth (Taurus, second house). There are many tendencies for alternate health issues in this birth chart, but for simplicity, we will use the teeth.

This child is raised on junk foods and soft drinks, exacerbating the natal potential. In his 7th year, in May, he begins complaining of severe toothache. This is shown by the *early trigger of the July progression* by the

## PROGRESSIONS WITH TRANSIT TRIGGERS

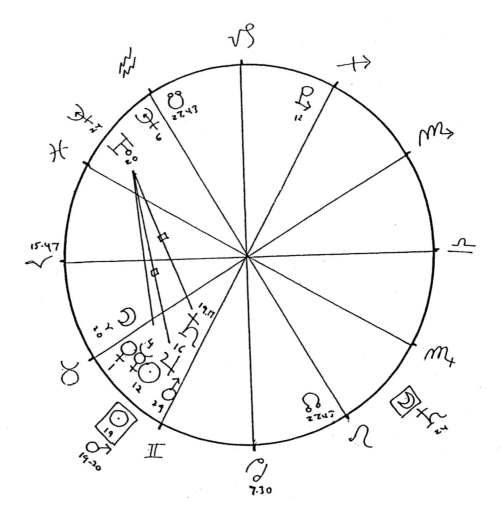

Inner Wheel: Natal Chart for May 2nd, 2000, 4 AM. *Dental issue.*

Boxed Sun and Moon in Outer Wheel: Progressions* at 7th year.
Only these two progressions are shown because they emphasize
the area near 19° Taurus, *the degree of natal Saturn.*

Outer Wheel (unboxed): Transits to July 3rd, 2007 (in the 7th year).
*Note:* Only the most important transit trigger planets are given. Notice, the
progressed Sun conjoins natal Saturn in the 7th year. Then, in July of the 7th
year, transit Mars conjoins both the progressed Sun and natal Saturn; while
transit Saturn squares this duo.

*Secondary Progressions* used. The Sun's position is the most important
progression of this system (one day of life equals one year of life). In this
figure, the progressed Sun achieves the degree of natal Saturn in the 7th year.

transit conjunction of the Sun plus the simultaneous square of transit Saturn in that month to the natal Saturn position in the sign of the teeth.

By July, the transiting conjunction of Mars to the the progressed Sun conjunct natal Saturn duo in Taurus coincides with major dental surgery to clean out infected teeth. It is a long and difficult surgery. Braces are also being discussed to correct an overbite.

This unfortunate tooth situation could have been minimized by proper adherence to tooth hygiene and diet prior to the "promised" date for onset. It also could have bounced to the ears, thyroid or neck, the other areas ruled by Taurus, or could have manifested as Leo (back, heart) or Scorpio (colon, genital) issues instead!

"Good grief!" you ask; "so how do you know which region is manifesting? Easy! *The client tells you!* Usually by this time, the native has clear cut symptoms. Your study of the chart at this point can target the true source of the problem. You may also discover clues for treatment and provide safer dates for the timing of treatment or surgery. (Chapter 23).

This brief sample should give you an idea how to work this system.

*Note: The Moon's crossing by hard aspect of the established problem degree(s) can time your layering of progressions and transits to a single day.*

## THE MOST IMPORTANT HEALTH TRANSITS

1) Any slower planet transiting a Lunar Node should signal your immediate attention. The natal North Node opens the door to potentially receiving an excess of that transiting planet's energy.

The natal South Node is a hole for the energy of the transiting plane's energy to drain out. Both conditions (planet transits of No. or So. Nodes) are common at the onset of serious diseases both mental or physical.

The natal South Node, being more negative, appears to be the most reliable. *Transiting* planets to *natal* nodes will act similarly as discussed in Chapter 11 for the *natal* conjunctions of planets with the *natal* Lunar Nodes.

2) Transit Saturn in hard aspect to the Sun reduces the Vital Force.

3) Transit Saturn in hard aspect to the Moon depresses the system and this is no time to fool lightly with your health and diet. Absorption of nutrients is lessened and the female system cooled. This is one testimony of menopause, should it occur in the appropriate age range. The emotional life and mind are profoundly effected in a lead like manner. Stimulants, warmth and good cheer are required.

4) Transit Saturn conjunct Venus reduces the female hormones and is one testimony of menopause if occurring in the appropriate age range. Transit Saturn conjunct Mars reduces the male hormones.

5) Transit Jupiter in hard aspect to Sun or Moon produces over extension of the vital forces and a disordered system. Temperance is required.

6) Transit Uranus crossing any planet disorders this planet and produces a nervous state. For instance, transit Uranus conjunct Mars produces a hyperactive state and insomnia. Transit Uranus conjoined Mercury produces nerve pains and mental trials (when negative.

7) Transit Neptune conjoined any planet will weaken or diffuse its natural force.

8) Slower planets crossing the ascendant may be strongly felt throughout the whole bodily system.

9) The transit South Node crossing the ascendant, or even in the ascending sign produces extreme fatigue. This reliable phenomenon is due to a form of astralic "leak" unknown to modern medicine. It is important to encourage extra Vital Force into the body through known methods such as pranayama or raw foods. Transit So. Node crossing any natal planet temporarily weakens the bodily function and/or region symbolized by that planet.

10) Transit Mars conjoined any planet heats up that planet. Transit Mars crossing the natal Moon or ascendant may signal an increased susceptibility to flu, rash, burns, or bacterial invasion.

11) Transit Saturn in the 6th house focuses one's attention on health. Neglected health issues may crop up during this transit.

12) Transit Saturn in the 8th sign as counted from the Ascendant as "1", counterclockwise, is the most important health transit of Saturn's house cycle. In these years one is provided the opportunity to renew, cleanse and transform oneself, or one will get worse. One must put oneself seriously to this task.

13) An eclipse occurring within 1° of the natal Sun is very profound, with effects (below) for at least three months, if not one year or more. Should the South Node be near the Sun, expect a "power outage" of Vital Force. This may result in reduced vitality, loss of ambition, spiritual urges, and in rare cases presents a threat to life. The body parts governed by the sign the power outage occurs in may weaken or fail. Protective thoughts and strategies are encouraged.

If the North Node is near the Sun, expect a "power surge" within three months of a Solar eclipse. A cosmic power surge eclipse expresses itself as increased vitality, ambition, worldly connections. However, too much energy may enter the physical system in the body parts associated with either the sign, element or sign polarity of an eclipse. For instance, the risk of heart attacks increases substantially near North Node eclipses in the sign of Leo, ruling sign of the heart.

Eclipses of all types near the natal Sun's degree (Solar, Lunar, North Node and South Node) are dangerous should there be any extant delicacy in the body part governed by the sign of the natal Sun, or its opposite sign.

## THE DECUMBITURE

This term literally means a "lying down". Decumbitures establish the medical branch of Horary Astrology, the specialist art of interpreting question charts calculated for precise moments of time.

The Classical Western astrologers calculated a chart for the time the patient "took to his bed". This decumbiture was used for prognosis, the judgment of both length and severity of illness and also to find the "critical days", occurring when the Moon aspected her decumbiture degree by any division of the wheel by eight: 45°, 90°; 135°, 180°, 225°, 270°, or back to start at 0°.

Every 7th day was extremely critical and marked a change in affairs for good or ill, dependent on the Moon's aspects. These dates would coincide with the Moon's applying square, opposition, departing square or renewed conjunction with her decumbiture degree.

The decumbiture ascendant sign and degree were especially important towards evaluation of patient constitution, disease diagnosis and severity.

There were many other specialist rules of interpretation within this system not included here. The student interested in decumbiture technology is directed to make a study of Horary astrology, and also to to obtain a copy of *A Handbook of Medical Astrology* by Jane Ridder-Patrick. This book elucidates the details of this ancient system of decumbiture to perfection, also providing a highly useful chapter on individual degrees.

In pre-modern times when the natal chart was rarely available, the calculation of the decumbiture was standard practice. It remains a valuable tool, but should never upstage the testimonies of the natal chart, should such be obtainable. Best results are obtained by studying the natal predispositions, the current progressed and transit "triggers", and then observing a decumbiture for diagnostic confirmation, bodily part emphasis and the establishment of critical days.

For instance, if your natal chart suggests two or three possible signs of the disease causation, the rising sign of the decumbiture can be your tie breaker.

*Note:* Most patients today to not write down the exact minute they took to their beds (did they ever?). They may not even take to their beds! Therefore, it is typically impossible to calculate a useful decumbiture.

**Strictures Against Judgment of the Decumbiture**

In Horary Astrology, all question charts, including the Decumbiture should not be interpreted should the following conditions apply:

1) The ascendant is between 1-3° of a sign, unless the querent is a child (too early to pose a question.)

2) The ascendant is between 27-30° of a sign (too late to ask the question).

3) Moon "void of course", i.e. making no further aspects to any planet before leaving the sign. Some astrologers do not feel Luna is void if she accomplishes a parallel of declination with another planet. A void-of-course Moon indicates the question is void, going nowhere and therefore your answer will somehow come to naught. It is possible that this rule would not apply for decumbitures.

4) The Moon is in the Via Combusta: 15° Libra through 15° Scorpio. This was considered so evil in Horary that one must avoid reading the chart entirely.
  This rule, though traditional, seems an odd one. There are many "evil" degrees scattered throughout zodiac and modern astrologers do not corroborate an exceptional evil to this entire area from the last half of Libra through the first half of Scorpio. In fact, the sweetest star in the heavens, blessed Spica, is located herein, in late Libra. Could it be that this area once proved a doozie for some ancient astrologer's client and he passed this "rule"

down to us as unfailing tradition?

5) Saturn is in the 7th house (the astrologer will err in judgment).

6) Ruler of the 7th house is debilitated (i.e. in detriment or fall positions) or retrograde (faulty judgment).

7) Saturn is in the ascendant, especially if retrograde. (A bad start for the whole chart.) However, this position may remain useful for medical Horary because Saturn rising at the time of the decumbiture would certainly describe a compromised condition of the querent, and something about the health condition.

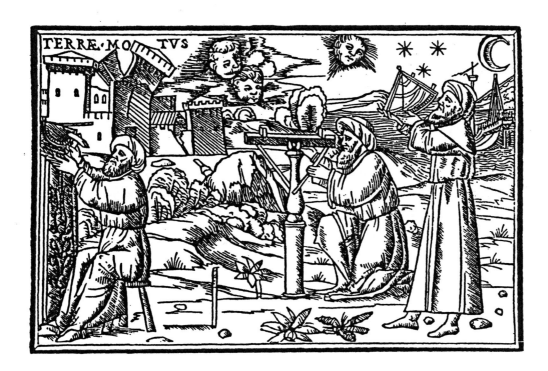

# Astro-Diagnosis

It may be illegal in your state or country to diagnose or to give medical advice of any kind without a license in medicine. Please study the example disclaimer form for providing surgery dates in Chapter 22. This book includes no disclaimer form for providing readings in Medical Astrology because you can not legally do so anyway at this time.

What you can do is give a lesson in Classical Western medical astrology, using the client's chart as a hypothetical example. The reading of the client's birth chart is to be viewed and stated as an interesting educational experience and not medical practice. It must be very carefully explained to your client that you are not a licensed medical practitioner (unless you are), nor is not legal for you to diagnose or give advice, and furthermore, that any ideas they obtain from the reading should never be acted upon without the opinion of a qualified medical practitioner.

And do not be a fool. If you are going to provide medical astrology services it is important that you know basic anatomy and the symptoms of basic problems.

But for your own interest, how would you begin a diagnosis should someone you know get sick? First, note the date or general time the problem began. Make a thorough inquiry as to the exact nature of the complaint. Let us say your spouse announces one morning:

"I am getting nauseous after eating fried eggs".

OK, now what? In your mental bank, you should have some idea of several possible causes for nausea after ingesting eggs. Some of these are: toxic liver, obstructed gall bladder, parasites in the gall ducts, parasites or worms in the intestines or colon, stomach ulcer, imbalance or change in stomach enzymes and acids, gas, blood poisoning from the eggs, virus, emotional problems associated with eggs.

Start asking questions. Find out as much as you can about attendant symptoms, and the precise location and sensation of the "stomach nausea". (A surprising number of people mistake their intestine for their "stomach").

Now in this same mental bank of yours you have a clear idea of what signs and planets govern which organs. All of that information is found in the preceding chapters.

You now proceed to scan the chart for any planets, especially malefics or the Moon, in the signs of the stomach, liver or intestine. Lo and behold, you discover a natal emphasis in Virgo ( the intestines, pancreas, appendix, liver), but no natal planet in Cancer (the sign that rules the stomach). You also find that Jupiter (the liver) is at its "fall" in Virgo, retrograde, and near the Lunar South node, thus gravely weakened.

Now check the timing of onset. Perhaps the recent eclipse just squared the location of this Jupiter. Or maybe transit Saturn is conjunct or opposing natal Jupiter.

If so, you can suspect a torpid liver, and not the suggested stomach is the true cause of the nausea, encouraged by the fact that it was the fatty fried eggs that set off the nausea.

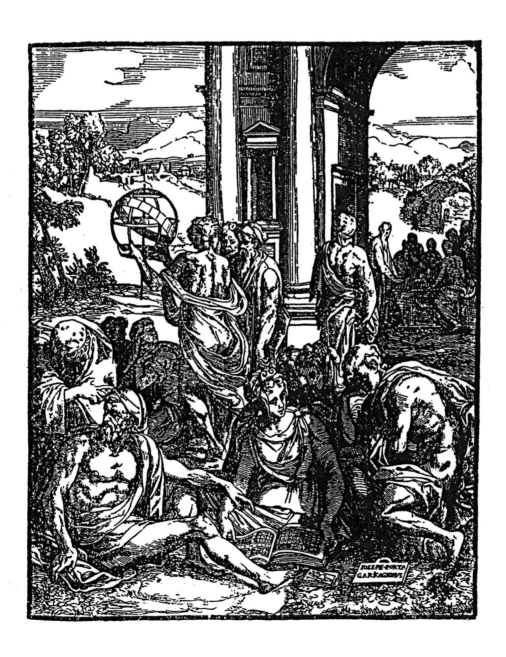

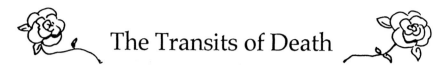 The Transits of Death

Yes, death can sometimes be predicted to the day. I've seen it myself several times. But let us emphasize the word *sometimes*. Transits indicating death may work out in all kinds of interesting ways and it is not the astrologer's province to be certain of any aspect meaning death.

Despite death transits, modern medicine steps in to save many a "death". My favorite example was that of a man whose chart demonstrated several of the classical transits of death all colluding on the same date. Of course, I said nothing. The deadly date arrived and he proceeded to have heart failure and died. However, a medical team resuscitated him with the latest equipment and he went on to win awards in his field, making his wife very happy.

There are those who state that your time of death is immutable. Perhaps this is true in some cases, but certainly not all. The Hindu idea seems more realistic: that karma and destiny is fixed for some individuals, whereas for others it is flexible, and then there are those cases in between!

Of course, the question remains: "Should the astrologer predict death?" To predict death would seem unethical in most cases. You, the astrologer, might see in a chart what you think may be death but are wise to keep quiet about it. There is no need to senselessly frighten your client or hapless friend!

In very rare cases you may be asked to give your opinion on the general time of death in a hopelessly terminal case. Such information might be very useful to the individual although I will leave this matter between you, him/her; their God and your own good conscience.

So why know the *Transits of Death?* These are very important to know indeed!

Armed with this knowledge you might forestall what otherwise would be a death or serious illness. Like anything else in life, sometimes it is only a matter of "forewarned is forearmed." Do not suggest to a client with severe bowel troubles that death looks imminent, but rather perhaps to get that exploratory colonoscopy before their three month trip to Bali!

Below, is a list of some of the more important aspects that occur near the death of an individual. Normally, several *testimonies* of death are required, and the background *progressions* must agree.

You will notice that most of these fatal transits are from planets, nodes and eclipses to the natal Sun, Moon or ascendant. This is because the degrees of these three natal points are the "givers of life" or *anaretic degrees.*

Most frequently occurring death aspects are from the transiting malefics and/or eclipses in hard aspect or quincunx to these three life points.

*Dear Reader, please be strongly reminded that you, your friends and family will all experience all of the below transits multiple times in a lifetime WITHOUT DYING. Please do not think "oh my God, Saturn is conjunct my Sun therefore I am about to die!!!" It takes several strong aspects to cook the goose, astrologically speaking. These aspects are most useful when charting a terminal illness or someone at the extremity of old age.*

TRANSITS OF DEATH
*(Warning: Do not enter here without first reading the above paragraph!)*

1) Transit Saturn conjunct or oppose the natal Sun within a few degrees. Saturn usually makes this "pass" three times and is most powerful when *retrograde* or *stationary.*

2) Transit Saturn square the natal Sun (weaker than the above two).

3) An eclipse within 1° of the natal Sun. The South Node near the Sun is more powerful than the North Node. (One of the Nodes is always near the eclipsed point!) The eclipse date is not necessarily an event date as the eclipse effect may span three months to a year, waiting to "hatch" when triggered by other transits.

Following the eclipse, look for dates the transit Sun or Mars arrives by conjunction, square or opposition to the degree of the eclipse. Transiting South Node crossing the natal Sun much weakens the vitality.

4) An eclipse within 1° of the natal Moon. The South Node style eclipse near the Moon is more negative than the North Node type eclipse near the Moon. Transiting South Node crossing the natal Moon exhausts the native. The eclipse date is not necessarily an event date as the eclipse effect may span three months to a year, waiting to "hatch" when triggered by transits.

*Mark those dates within the year when the transit Sun or Mars arrives by conjunction, square or opposition to the degree of the eclipse.*

5) Natal ascendant ruler transiting the 8th house and conjunct a malefic.

6) Transit Saturn in quincunx (150°) of natal Sun, Moon or ascendant by one degree.

7) Transit Saturn transiting through the 8th sign of the birth map, counting from the ascendant as "1", counterclockwise.

8) Transit Saturn crossing the natal South Lunar Node.

9) Transit Saturn crossing the descendant point (opposite the ascendant). Of the four angles, the descendant is the most death oriented. As the preeminent life timing device, Saturn is frequently seen transiting any one of the four natal angles at the time of death, including the descendant. Saturn crossing an angle marks an important life juncture as follows: the *ascendant:* "old life ends, new life chapter begins"; the *nadir:* "endings"; the *descendant:* "setting, pause point in life, point where the Sun sets"; the *midheaven:* "achievement, finalization of accomplishment, the peak".

10) For Jupiterian diseases, Jupiter squaring or opposing the Sun is especially dangerous. Should the Ascendant be Virgo or Capricorn, and the native suffer from any Jupiterian complaint, then the period of Jupiter's transit passage through these signs is dangerous.

11) Jupiter transiting the 8th sign from the ascendant counting counterclockwise. Count the ascendant sign as "1".

12) Transit Jupiter *quincunx* (150°) the natal Sun within one degree. This is dangerous if the Sun simultaneously receives a conjunction, square, opposition or quincuncx aspect of Saturn; or a conjunction or square from the South Node.

13) Transit Jupiter *quincunx* (150°) of the natal Moon within one degree. This is dangerous in lunar diseases, or if the Moon is "hyleg", (see below). Observe if the Moon simultaneously receives a dangerous aspect from transit Saturn or the South Node. *Note: Transit Jupiter is more problematic for Virgo, Gemini and Capricorn Ascendants. Also, this transit has a marked effect on the mental health, placing the mind under unusual strain.*

14) For Virgo, Capricorn or Gemini ascendants, the passage of transit

Jupiter over the ascendant can be dangerous if the native suffers from a Jupiter - related ailments such as diabetes, liver problems or obesity.

15) Transiting Jupiter conjunct the natal South Lunar Node.

16) Curiously, Jupiter, our great benefic, is often seen transiting a natal angle at the time of death. Because Jupiter is thought to govern the spirit body, could this transit bring release?

17) A South Node - style eclipse occurring within three degrees over the birth ascending degree.

18) Transit Mars conjunct or oppose the natal Sun. This transit is more powerful if retrograde or stationary. The square is also dangerous if the individual is already ill.

19) Transit Mars conjunct or oppose the natal Moon. Most powerful when retrograde or stationary. The square is also dangerous.

20) Transit Mars conjunct the natal South Node.

21) Transit Mars in a close quincunx (150°) to natal Sun, Moon or ascending degree.

22) Uranus is involved in sudden, unexpected death, often seen in close conjunction with Jupiter, either Lunar Node, or the lights (Sun or Moon).

23) Exact or close conjunctions of transiting Saturn, Uranus, Neptune and Pluto with each other's natal positions is very frequent.

24) The Nodal Return and the Nodal Reverse are not uncommon transits at the time of death.

25) The Hyleg (page 112 - usually the natal Sun or Moon) positioned in the *bends*, or between the transiting nodes exactly.

# The Houses of Life and Death

**Classical Life Giving Regions of the Birth Chart termed the** *Aphetic* **zones.**
*Note:* Use the ascendant degree as your starting point.

• 25th degrees of the "8th house" to the 25th degree of the "11th house". Best results are obtained by using the 25th degree of the 8th *sign* to the 25th degree of the 11th *sign* as counted from the ascendant degree as "0°", counterclockwise.

• The 25th degree of the 12th sign to the 25th degree of the 1st sign (as above).

• The 25th degree of the 6th sign to the 25th degree of the 7th sign.

**All remaining regions of the birth chart are termed** *Anaretic,* **or taking of life. Transiting planets are more dangerous when traveling through the** *Anaretic* **regions.**

FINDING THE "HYLEG", THE PLANETARY GIVER OF LIFE.

**Males:** Traditionally, the natal Sun is *Hyleg* if located in one of the *Aphetic* regions above. If the Sun is not found to be in an *Aphetic* zone, use natal Jupiter or the natal Moon.
*Note*: Another term for *Hyleg* is the *Apheta.*

**Females:** Traditionally, the natal Moon is *Hyleg*, or the *Apheta* if located in an *Aphetic* region. If Luna is not found in an *Aphetic* zone, use natal Venus. If Venus is not aphetic, use the Ascendant degree. (See note, below!)

**Important Note for Female Charts:**
Personally, the author has not found a huge difference between male and female charts at the time of death. In her experience, ascendant and Sun seem equally important for both genders. Notice how Sol is not even listed as a *Hyleg* for females, an oversight that seems preposterous.
A woman's natal Sun is often severely afflicted in crises or death

and we would be foolish indeed to ignore this fact in favor of ancient gender - based *Hyleg* doctrine. It is not understood why tradition applies Venus greater powers of life over females than Sol, our very center of Vital Force!

Natal Jupiter seems equally aphetic for both genders at the time of death. (Jupiter has a strong affinity with the spirit body, which knows no gender!)

Other ancient systems might lend the Sun a greater candidacy for *Hyleg* in day births for either gender, and the Moon in the case of night births.

Perhaps this curious Venus association with female life an death was due to the fact that until modern times the rate of women dying from Venus-Moon associated childbirth, was often as high as 25%! It is important to question certain traditions that may owe more to culture, historical environment or theory than to reality.

However, no true systematic research has been accomplished on this interesting subject of gender associated Hylegs and death. The jury is out, so you must see for yourself if the tradition holds true!

TIPS ON DEATH TRANSITS

Potentially death dealing transits are much stronger if afflicting the natal planets out of *anaretic* regions (above).

The most dangerous situation to observe is a negative health aspecting planet out of an anaretic region afflicting the *Hyleg*, which is always located in an *aphetic* region. (Any other natally afflicted planet could be in any region. However, the *Hyleg*, or giver of life, by its' very definition must stand in an aphetic region. See above.)

There are three preeminent transit planets that may signify death when transiting relevant positions in the natal chart: transit Saturn, transit Mars, and the transiting ruler of the individual's personal natal chart's 8th sign (as counted from the ascendant sign as "1", counterclockwise).

The *natal* positions of the death dealing planets Mars and Saturn were known *Anaretic promittors*, because they promised death and brought that promise to pass. A *promittor* is a natal planet to which any progressed *significator* (of any astrological house and its' issues) moves to aspect by progression. The aspect delivers the "promise". Please remember that one receives hundreds of negative aspects to one's promittors during one's lifetime without dying.

# Treatment Types by Planet

Every natal or transit planet in excess can be antidoted by the remedies of the traditionally balancing planet. Conversely, a planetary deficiency may be remedied by applying treatments encouraging more of the weak planet's natural energy. Below is a brief outline of remedials followed by the system of planetary antidotes.

**Sun:** Heat. The Sun. Pranic healing. Orange or golden light. Enzymes, Light therapy. Laser?

**Moon:** Fluids, water treatment (magnetized water), hydrotherapy, hydration, nutritives, demulcents, liquid diet.

**Mercury:** Mental and physical exercise that stimulates the nerves and coordination. Speech therapy. Breathing therapies. Cognitive therapies and analysis, journaling, nutrition. The study of health and nutrition are Mercurial interests. Hatha Yoga?

**Venus:** Soothing, relaxing remedies. Massage, aromatherapy, pleasure, sedatives, anodynes, flower essences (with Neptune).

**Mars:** Muscular aerobic exercise, iron, heat, counterirritation, emetics, purgatives, rolfing, meat eating, surgery, lancing, acupuncture (with Uranus, Neptune and Pluto) movement therapies, Pilates, martial arts, sweating, stimulants, rubefacients, stimulating massage, diaphoretic herbs, diuretics, antiseptics.

**Jupiter:** Attention to correct type and balance of fats. External application of oils. Aligning one's lifestyle and diet to appropriate medical philosophies (yoga etc.), health philosophy, appeals to a higher power, Medical Astrology, prayer, golden light visualization, intervention by saints or angelic beings.

**Saturn:** Cold packs, braces and casts, chiropractic work, mineral therapies, fasting, weightlifting, styptics, astringents, retirement from society, celibacy, abstinence from certain activities or foods, clay treatments, febrifuges.

Saturn is the balance wheel of the planets (Saturn is exalted in

Libra, the sign of the scales). In palmistry, the Saturn finger balances the entire hand. He is capable of antidoting more of the planetary conditions than any other planet.

•The cold nature of Saturn antidotes heated Mars or Sun conditions.

•Saturn's astringency is useful for Jupiter's over expansion, Mars' bleeding or the atonic ailments of Venus, South Node or Neptune.

•A disciplinarian, Saturn's wisdom and restraint antidotes the indulgences of Venus, Neptune and Mars.

•A monkish planet, his cures and color (deep blue) are useful for the scattered nerves of Mercury. Earthy Saturn's steadiness and grounding ability antidotes Uranus' electrical extremes.

**Uranus:** Electricity (see works of Edgar Cayce on wet cell appliance, violet ray, etc.), oscillation therapies, radionics. Vibration therapies (with Neptune), medical astrology, sonar therapy? See Neptune.

**Neptune:** Sleep, sonar therapy, aromatherapy, homeopathy, flower essences, the ocean, soporifics, anodynes, anaethesea, opiates, foot massage, hypnosis, suggestion, spiritual healing, Reiki (Neptune dominates the birth charts of many Reiki Masters), radionics and vibration therapies, medical psychism, prayer.

**Pluto:** Blood transfusion. Marrow transfusion. Organ transplant. Genetic therapies. Nuclear medicine. Radiation, chemotherapy, pro-biotics, antibiotics, gender reassignment.

## ANTIDOTES:

**Sun:** Discords of the Sun should be treated by antidoting the planets in disharmonious aspects to the Sun, rather than the Sun itself (Paul Bergner). One might also check the *element* of the natal Sun, and consider its' excesses in Chapter 15, if this applies. Should the natal Sun be too hot and dry, antidote with Saturn treatments (cold), or Moon remedies (moist and cool).

**Moon:** The Moon is cold, moist and fluidic. Traditionally, she is antidoted by the treatments of hot, stimulating Mars. However, the Lunar conditions of mental and emotional instability benefit from the stabilizing treatments of Saturn. Should the disharmonious Moon indicate nutritive insufficiency, then balance with Saturnian mineral treatments.

**Mercury:** Fidgety, nervous Mercury conditions benefit by ingestion of nervines (herbs that strengthen and tonify the nerves). Tension problems associated with Mercury can be soothed with Venus and Neptune treatments. Unstable, unfocused conditions of Mercury might benefit from the steadying application of Saturnian treatments. Always suspect mercury poisoning should an afflicted Mercury coincide with known symptoms of this ailment.

**Venus:** Relaxive, atonic conditions of Venus are traditionally benefited by astringent and strengthening Saturn treatments. Mars can also antidote Venus because aerobic, muscular activity antidotes sluggishness and also Mars' acid provides the perfect balance to Venus' alkalinity.

**Mars:** An overheated, dry Mars is traditionally antidoted by a cooling, moist Moon treatment. Moon treatments (ointments, demulcents, juices, salves) are best for hot, dry, itchy Mars problems. Saturn treatments apply the cold, styptic or restriction useful in Martian sprains or bleeding. The discipline and nutritives of Saturn strengthen a weak Mars as no other planet can. Saturn and Mars work together to build muscle. Astringent Saturn can also bind an excess release of toxins due to an overactive Mars.

**Jupiter:** Mercury treatments are traditionally assigned to antidote Jupiterian ailments. This is puzzling. Perhaps the Mercurial study of health, diet and nutrition antidote Jupiter's tendency toward obesity; or maybe Mercury's mercantile tendencies balance Jupiter's grandiosity. Saturnian fasting balances the overextended Jupiterian complaints such obesity or torpid liver.

**Saturn:** The relaxing treatments of Venus are traditionally useful for tense, stiff or just plain "uptight" Saturnian conditions. The heat of Mars antidotes Saturn's chilly stiffness. Mars' stimulating and blood cleansing qualities help offset Saturn's poor circulation and trend toward toxic buildup. Jupiter's oil treatments provide the lubrication necessary for preventing the onset of Saturn's rheumatic tendencies.

**Uranus:** There is as yet no established "traditional" antidote for Uranian conditions. Because of Uranus' electrical nature, it would be suggested that Saturn's grounding treatments be applied. The correct salts and minerals would be quite important (Saturn). *continued*

Venusian treatments might prove relaxing to the spasmodic problems of this planet and of course potassium/magnesium and calcium balances should be attended to.

**Neptune:** As yet, there is no traditionally established antidote for Neptunian conditions. Neptune's influence is ungrounded, responding well to quiet "reality" therapies such as gardening. Therefore, the earthy Saturnian treatments would seem a good antidote for the bohemian excesses of Neptune. The stimulating and iron enriching treatments of Mars might also be called for. Neptune, working through the subtle bodies, may respond to its own remedies best: homeopathy, music and/or, psychic intuition, hypnotic suggestion (very dangerous).

**Pluto:** Traditional antidotes to Plutonian problems have not been established. Pluto is very extreme in nature (boiling hot or frigid cold) producing drastic conditions that require radical solutions. Bergner sights Mars treatments as useful (purging, bacterial supplementation). Currently, Plutonian conditions appear to be treated with Pluto's remedies: Nuclear medicine, laser surgery, chemotherapy, organ transplantation, gender reassignment. Laser?

## VEDIC GEM PRESCRIPTIONS: "UPAYE".

The astrologers of India have a useful system of gem remedials for planetary problems. The West, once possessing similar remedials, seems to have laid them aside somewhere in favor of psychological astrology, discoveries of new planets, and all manner of astrological innovations. This section is included for those who wish to study this ancient system of gem remedials.

There are many other forms of planetary remedials including: ceremonies, change of name, chants, and charity. All the above methods aim at altering the pattern one is projecting into the universe. In essence, the idea is to change one's vibrational resonance and thus cease attracting types of events or illnesses particular to one's set resonance pattern and internal time clock.

What is the technology behind Vedic gem prescriptions? We can expand this question by asking "What is the technology behind amulets and talismans of any kind?" Generally, amulets and talismans work through at least five different technologies! Most such devices use only one or two.

These methods are both practical and magical. Any device designed to adjust one's subtle energies would be "practical". Any device that works exclusively through thought power, or by means of attracting the assistance of outside entities or thought forms (such as magic sigils) would be seen here as "magical".

The attraction of outside entities is not advised. We never know the true nature and intent of such entities! However, the use of gems as practical devices is no different from wearing an orthodic in your shoe for a foot problem - provided you can correctly prescribe!

In *Upaye*, or the method of Vedic gem prescriptions, use is made of both the practical and the magical. However, the upaye system works very well with no use of the magical whatever.

HOW GEM REMEDIES WORK  (various metaphysical technologies)
1) attract more of a  desired planet's energy. For example, should we not receive enough of the Sun's energy, we can correct this deficit by bringing more Sun energy to our subtle and physical bodies by wearing the Sun's gem red ruby.

2) Antidote, or adjust an excessive amount of a select planet's energy. Example: Should we, at birth, be out of whack with Saturn, then perhaps a gem correction could act like a lens to harmonize the incoming rays of this planet.

3) Gems can also be used to  deflect  negative energies (the umbrella technique). As an aside, Chinese Feng Shui practitioners make ample use of mirrors for both deflection of negative energies, absorption of good energies, and magnification of desired energies (as you desire!)

4) Absorb negative energies. Opaque minerals like malachite and turquoise are very useful absorbatives and physical body protectors.

5) Carry imprinted intent. In the Vedic system all remedial gems are imprinted ceremonially with a specific healing intent before wearing. A strong thought is placed upon the gem through purification, chanting and other methods. We do know that crystals are natural radio receivers so crystalline gems are especially useful for this purpose.

**The Effect of Color**
The energy of planets in your chart is either enhanced, reduced or

harmonized primarily through use of color, and only secondarily, the gem. To wear *red* attracts more of Sun and Mars. *Emerald green is* for Mercury, *transparent white* attracts Venus, *yellow* for Jupiter, *orange* for North Lunar Node, *dark blue* for Saturn, *white* for Moon, and dual colored stones for the South Lunar Node (like cat's eye).

Those who can't afford gems can substitute stones of colored glass or even drink bottles of colored water. However, the actual gem has a distinct influence of its own, and it is of course preferable to use the expensive gem over glass!

### Traditional Vedic Gem-Planet Associations

The traditional Vedic gem-planet associations are as follows:
Sun-*red ruby* or substitute red garnet; Moon-*pearl* or substitute moonstone; Mercury-*green emerald* or substitute green tourmaline; Venus-*white diamond,* or substitute zircon or rock crystal; Mars-*red coral;* Jupiter-*yellow sapphire,* or substitute yellow citrine, yellow zircon; Saturn-*blue sapphire,* or substitute lapis lazuli; North Node-*gomedha;* South Node-*cat's eye.*

Vedic gems are never worn without proper ceremony. This ceremony acts to attract and imbue further energies into the gem, in what might be termed a *thought form impression.* For instance, various chants to the planetary deity are amply used. These practices qualify as religious and/or magical.

Such ceremonies are thought to create a very powerful effect in the prescribed jewelry. It is also true that on a purely practical level, a correctly prescribed gem can be powerful through the adjustments it naturally brings to one's energy fields. One does not need to be a religious Hindu to benefit from a gem's practical corrective effects.

The traditional Upaye system is cook-book in approach, with extensive ritual detail. The bibliography references three excellent books that define this system's rules and rituals in detail.

However, I will give the basic rules here: Planets that govern the "good" houses 1, 5 and 9 are definitely safe to strengthen by wearing their associated gem. If these planets are already in good shape, the gem is not necessary, but will increase the good fortune anyway. If the planetary ruler of one of these houses is weak or afflicted, then wearing their gem will act to either partially or totally correct the problem.

The planetary rulers of the "evil" *dusthana* houses 6, 8 and 12 are not wise to strengthen, even if they appear to need it. The idea being that enhancing these planets enhances your bad luck! Being a Vedic system, the Vedic zodiac is used. There are several Vedic zodiacal wheels to select from, varying from 1-6 degrees in difference between them.

# How to Find a Safe Surgery Date

This fascinating chapter includes the following sections: Basics, Intake, Client's Contract, Tools/House Systems, Medical Rulerships by sign/house, Bodily systems (the 6 sign polarities), Body parts ruled by the Planets, Pathological Action of the Planets, Lights and Nodes, Surgery Rules - dos and don'ts, Electional Suggestions, Let's Read Charts! - Surgery Examples, The Electional Chart. The following chapter includes two example surgeries from the astrological view: a face lift and a knee replacement.

**Basics:**

To find a safe surgery date, it is important to first establish your "intake". Ask your client the following questions, below. His/Her answers are essential because without them you will not properly understand the case. Surgery is a life/death matter. You must take your work with surgery electionals very seriously. Write the answers down and make sure you understand the surgery date request and your client's case thoroughly.

## Intake:

1. What part of the body, exactly, is to be operated upon and why?
2. Does the operation involve removal or addition of material from/to the body?
3. Where is the surgery to take place (what city)?
4. Is this surgery optional or mandatory?
5. If optional surgery, then what are your preferential time parameters (months, days, etc.)?
6. If non optional surgery, then what are your maximum time boundaries?
7. What dates and times is the surgeon restricted to?
8. Was there a date the problem began?
9. What could go wrong in this kind of surgery you will be having?
10. Has this body part been operated on before? If so, when?
11. If the body part has been previously operated on, was it successful or not? What happened? What was the date? Check the transits on that date.
12. Can you obtain the surgeon's birth data, or at least his/her date and year of birth? (optional)
13. What is the client's birth date, time, place and year? (essential)

## Client's Contract

It is important to protect yourself from any blame or dissatisfaction resulting from a surgery you have timed. Therefore, draw up a form similar to the following example form or best, have a lawyer design it. Your client signs it prior to beginning work on timing his/her surgery date.

I, _____, hereby understand that _____ is providing me, in return for an agreed payment, with an astrological opinion regarding an appropriate date and/or time for my surgery. I understand that_____ is not a medical authority and that the opinion on surgical timing obtained is not a medical opinion. I will not hold the below signed astrological timing consultant in any way responsible for the outcome of surgery or for my satisfaction with surgical results. I have provided the below signed astrological consultant with the necessary time parameters obtaining to this surgical procedure as suggested to me by my doctor or surgeon. My surgical time parameters are: _____
Signed_____ (client) Astrological Consultant_____
(you) Date_____

## Tools For Selecting Safe Surgery Dates.

A clean copy of the client's birth chart, plus current transits and progressions for the client. The chart must be very clear. *Remove excessive asteroids.* It is suggested that you have as simple a chart as possible. Be sure to include both lunar nodes.

If obtainable, the chart of the date of the accident or onset of problem is useful for identifying the focal planet(s) and sign relevant to the case.

A chart of the surgeon's birth day and year (birth time usually unobtainable) is useful to have on hand. A firm knowledge of body parts and their astrological rulerships (a limited list is given below.)

A firm general knowledge of medical astrology and/or medicine will be a real plus. One should have memorized the pathological action of each planet, and know the bodily rulerships for all planets, signs and houses.

## House System:

Whole sign houses are suggested. Alternative: work with the system you prefer, but do read natal and transit planetary aspects of 150° to the natal ascendant as stressful and critical. Also, for medical purposes, do consider any planet located in the natal 6th, 8th or 12th signs from the ascendant, (counting clockwise, ascendant as "1") as behaving as if in those houses.

**Essential Books:**

*The Encyclopedia of Medical Astrology* by H. L. Cornell, M. D. If you are serious astrologer and plan to select electional charts for surgery dates, then please invest in a copy of this amazing medical tome. If you are already familiar with medical rulerships you can go directly to Surgery Rules. The astro-medical rulerships by sign and house given in previous chapters are absolutely essential to know. It goes without saying that you must be familiar with traditional rulerships of the body: by planet, house and sign.

Remember, the planet acts upon the sign, and less so the other way around! *Example*: Mars heats up Cancer (the stomach), so you get ulcers; but watery, Moon-ruled Cancer does not necessarily cool off Mars so as to produce a lack of digestive acid. However, there are occasional exceptions to this rule. Mars is altered by the sign Cancer: he turns inward and goes defensive instead of aggressive. But he is still Mars! And he still applies his inflaming rays to the body parts governed by this sign.

**Surgery Rules**

Below is a list of most glaring "don'ts", and most obvious "dos". Still, your own intuition and expertise must be applied. Keep in mind that optional surgery is a very different matter than mandatory surgery. Those dangerous transits holding sway just prior, or during emergency situations could be fatal should one NOT operate. If this is the case, you must still attempt to dodge the worst aspects, or set a surgery date prior to their onset if at all possible.

## DON'TS: AVOIDING SURGICAL NIGHTMARES

1) Do not operate if the Moon is transiting the sign ruling the body part to be operated upon.

*Note*: this widely respected rule is not impervious. I have seen cases when a very nicely aspected Moon transiting through the sign of the operated body part coincided with a perfect surgery.

Ptolemy (140 A.D., *Tetrobiblios*) adds to this famous rule that one can IDEALLY give health treatments when the Moon is in the sign of the body part to be treated, but never, never, never to "pierce with iron" that same body part! The pull of the Moon could cause excessive swelling or bleeding in the body region of the Moon's transiting sign, especially at full Moon.

2) **Never operate if transit Mars is conjunct either the natal or transit South Lunar Node.** The natal South Node is the more important.

How close? That depends. For expected long recoveries, the transit Mars should avoid even the sign of the natal South Node. THIS IS A PRIMARY RULE. Ideally, no transiting planets or lights (Sun and Moon), should be journeying within three degrees of the natal South Node! This is not always avoidable, but do try! The approach of Mars to the South Node is worse than his departure, but never sanction elective surgery unless Mars is well clear of the South Node and no eclipse is upcoming within the month.

3) Do not operate if the most recent or soon upcoming eclipse was/is within three degrees of the natal South Node.

4) Avoid, if possible, a transit quincunx (150° aspect) from any planet to *any* natal planet, especially so if occurring within and orb of one degree.

5) Transit Mars should not be conjunct the natal Sun or Moon within several degrees. If unavoidable, it is certainly better for Mars to separate than apply (do make sure he has separated by at least one full degree). The square and opposition of transit Mars are not recommended either, but the conjunction is the most dangerous.

6) It is best if transit Saturn and Jupiter are not closely conjunct, square or oppose the Sun, Moon or the planet indicating the problem to be operated upon. This is not always possible to avoid because it is at these times the symptoms kick up a notch, demanding solution. (Jupiter's conjunction can go either way, being either highly protective or exceptionally stressful. You must ascertain if Jupiter is a positive or negative influence for the native).

7) Do not operate within 24-48 hours of full Moons.

8) Do not operate in an "eclipse month", especially if the sign polarity of the eclipse represents the pathology (i.e. Leo-Aquarius for the heart). Most typically, two eclipses occur in a four week period, twice a year. A week before the first eclipse through a week following the second eclipse is crucial. Especially avoid operating within one day of eclipses, or between two eclipses. Again, one cannot always avoid this should surgery be mandatory and/or of an emergency nature.

9) Avoid surgery should transit Mars be exactly conjunct or oppose natal

Uranus or Neptune. The opposite (transit Uranus or Neptune, and also transit South Node conjunct natal Mars) can likewise be dangerous.

10) Avoid surgery altogether if your natal 8th house is particularly lousy. Try alternative methods.

11) Avoid surgery in general if you have malefics or poorly placed planets in your natal 8th house in hard aspect to the Sun, Moon, or planet representing the problem area. *Example*: a natal Uranus-South Node conjunction in the natal 8th house in Cancer, closely squaring the natal Moon would bode ill for breast augmentation!

12) Transit Mars should never be retrograde or surgery may need to be repeated.

13) *Retrograde Rules of Surgical Avoidance:*
Saturn should not be retrograde for bone surgery. Venus must not be retrograde for ovarian surgery, nor Mercury for neurological, or ear work. Retrograde Jupiter is inadvisable for liver surgery, etc. Know your astromedical rulerships!

14) Major significators, or the natal Ascendant ruler should not be transiting the *fatal* degrees, i.e. the degree of the natal nodes, mean and true. (Use the degree positions of both the mean and true nodes).

15) The transiting nodes should not square by one degree the natal Sun, Moon, or the natal significator of the surgery (such as Jupiter for liver surgery). This puts that planet in *the bends* - a highly stressful condition.

16) The reverse of rule (15), above, is also true - transit planets ruling the body part in question should not transit the midpoint of the *natal* nodes on the date of surgery, thus simultaneously squaring both natal nodes, placing the transiting planet in the stressful bends.

## DO: HOW TO SELECT AN EXCELLENT SURGERY DATE

1) Transit Mars represents the surgeon's knife. This planet should ideally trine or sextile the planet representing the medical problem.

2) Transit Mercury reflects the surgeon's dexterity, and should follow the

above rule for Mars.

3) It is ideal to have transit Mars, Mercury and Moon all sextile or trine each other and also the natal planetary significator to be "operated upon".

4) Natal Sun, Moon and ascendant should ideally be free of close hard transit aspects and quincunxes (not always possible.)

5) The transit Sun in the 1st, 5th and 9th signs from the ascendant gives vital force, especially if also in trine or sextile, even loosely, to natal Sun.

6) It is quite good for transit Jupiter to conjunct, trine or sextile the natal Sun, Moon, Ascendant, or natal surgery focus planet (such as natal Mars for vasectomy). However, the conjunction of transit Jupiter is unpredictable, sometimes malefic, and should be avoided altogether if in Earth signs.

7) Transit Venus conjunct Sun, Moon, Ascendant, or natal surgery focus planet is soothing and protective. But don't depend on trines and sextiles of Venus to be of much significance! Transit Venus in the 6th and 7th houses provides good assistance and more pleasant social conditions during surgery and recovery.

8) Transit North Node in the sign of the body part to be operated upon is a good testimony, provided no eclipses are occurring that month.

9) Transit planets near the North Node bode success, especially if occurring within the sign reflecting the body part under surgery. Still, do not operate close to actual eclipses. *Ignore this rule for North Node ruled conditions such as boils, blood clots and impactions.*

10) *Moon Phase:* Transit Moon should be decreasing, and preferably in the last quarter for surgeries where post operative swelling or infection is a concern. However, the two days just before and of the New Moon are not advised. Decreasing Moon phases are also best for removal of growths and tissue.

Transit Moon should be in the 1st quarter for surgeries where new tissue must take and hold. In this case you do want an "increasing" energy. Still, avoid late second quarter, full Moon and early third quarter.

For eye surgery, transit Moon should be increasing. However, avoid the Full Moon by one-two days, as above, due to the tendency to swelling.

Absolutely avoid two weeks before to two weeks after any eclipse for any surgery, and the period between two eclipses - especially in Fire signs for vision repair.

## Exact Times

Occasionally, your client is able to closely time the onset of surgery, especially for mole removals and the like. Below are some rules for exact timing of surgical procedures. An *electional* chart is selected using these guidelines. The electional chart is not a natal chart. Rather, it is a pre-selected chart of the transits timed for a specific purpose - in our case, surgery.

The below suggestions for surgery electionals may be used in conjunction with the transits to the natal chart. Ideal surgery dates look good both ways - the transits to the natal positions are good; and the transit planets to other transit planets ( the electional chart) are also positive. Such ideal dates are hard to find and not always possible. The ideal planetary conditions for surgical electionals below occur *transit to transit* (not transit to natal). Naturally, you will not be able to obtain all suggested conditions, so you do the best you can.

## Electional Chart Suggestions for Surgeries:

1) The transit ascendant ruler and Moon should n̲o̲t̲ be located 12, 6 or 8 signs away from the transit ascendant. (Count ascendant as "1").

2) The transit ascendant ruler and Moon should apply by sextile and trine to transit benefics (Venus, Jupiter).

3) The transit ascendant ruler and Moon should never apply by conjunction, square or opposition to transit malefics (Saturn, Mars, Uranus); nor conjoin or square the transit or natal South Node.

4) Benefics near the angles of by a few degrees in the chart for the time of surgery (the surgical election) are helpful.

5) Malefics on the angles by a few degrees in the chart for the time of surgery (the surgical election) are harmful.

6) Ideally, the planet ruler of the electional chart's 8th house should be in a harmonious aspect to the ruler of the 1st house, and/or benefics.

**7) Lunar Avoids for Electional Charts:**

Avoid the transit conjunction of the Moon with transit Mars or Saturn. Transit Moon in an applying conjunction with transit Jupiter can be dangerous, especially in Earth or Water signs! Avoid the transit of the Moon through the "critical" degrees (every 13 degrees beginning with 0° Aries), or when in occultation (exact conjunction by declination and longitude) with a fixed star of a notoriously evil nature. You will need a computer program to find the occultations.

8) It is helpful for the sign governing the body part under surgery to be receiving good aspects. At the time of surgery, it is ideal for transit Venus to be moving through this sign. A trine from transit Jupiter, Mars or Moon is also excellent. *For best results, Mars, representative of the surgeon's knife, must be in harmony with the sign of the body part he cuts.*

9) Preferably, transit Mars should not be retrograde.

10) The planet representing the medical problem should not, by transit, be retrograde or exactly square the Lunar Nodes.

*Example:* Saturn rules the bones and should not be retrograde at bone surgery. Neither at bone or teeth surgery should transit Saturn be exactly squaring either the natal or transit Lunar Nodes within one degree unless unavoidable.

11) Preferably, the transit Moon should be swift in daily motion.

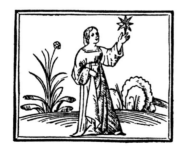

# Let's Do Surgery Charts

Ok, you've received your surgery chart selection basics. Now... Let's do Surgery Charts!

THE EXAMPLE CHARTS:
Charts are published without birth data to protect confidentiality. Transits are on outer wheel. We will not be using progressions in this lesson. We will not be engaged in timing surgery onset to the minute due to the futility of such attempts. (Surgery times routinely are delayed and are therefore out of the control of most clients.) *See exact timing tips, preceding.

CHART #1, page 130: *Face Lift.* Natal chart (inner wheel) with transits (outer wheel) for a "miraculously successful" face lift. Even the doctor was amazed at the fast healing and low scarring!

CASE OVERVIEW
This is a facelift, an elective operation of beautification (Venus) for the region of the face: observe Aries (upper face) and Taurus (for lower face and neck); 1st house (head and face).

Client preferred to have the operation somewhere between September and November of 1986. What do we do first? First we check for the existence of natal planets in Aries, Taurus or the 1st house. We discover a Jupiter-Uranus conjunction in early Aries. Early Aries governs the crown of the head, so will be less emphasized than one might think for a face lift. However, we should keep an eye to clear this area of stressful aspects, and fortify it, if possible.

Something should right away grab our attention. Wow! Here is natal Venus (beauty) and Mars (surgery) joined at the ascendant (face). We now know that this area MUST be fortified and MUST receive the trine or sextile of transit Mars, the surgeon's knife. Ideally, the transit Moon (flow of the day) and transit Mercury (surgeon's dexterity) should also trine or sextile to this combination.

THE SURGERY CHART #1 *Facelift Surgery*

Transit Mars and Moon would both be trining the natal Venus-Mars conjunct natal Ascendant (the face). Also, the transit Moon was in Taurus, a great sign for beauty. Although Taurus does indeed rule the lower face and neck, I ignored Ptolemy's rule of "pierce not" the body part ruled by the sign the transit Moon transits.

Why ignore the rule? Because not only is the transit Moon ideally aspected in a grand trine with transit Mars and natal Venus-Mars-Asc.; but is simultaneously in the 9th sign from the ascendant - one of the best and most vital, lucky houses. Also, a fixity of Taurus would seem ideal for a face lift. (Note: Vivien Robson, in *Electional Astrology*, suggests a Fixed Moon sign as best for surgery, although I would disagree with including the Fixed sign Aquarius - this sign being too disturbing on the electrical body).

Transit Mars is also in a life giving area - the 5th sign from the ascendant, and very powerful and consistent in Capricorn, the sign of Mars' exaltation. Thus, the transit Moon and Mars are simultaneously strong in the electional chart for the day, regardless of our client; and also in positive aspect to the facial part of the client's natal chart (asc). No serious "don'ts", (as listed earlier in the preceding article), are occurring on this day.

The natal Jupiter- Uranus planets in Aries (head) receive a stabilizing trine from transit Saturn. There is a close quincunx from transit Mars to natal Moon. Still, it is two degrees away, "dodging the bullet" of the stressful one degree quincunx. Why else did I go ahead? Because the transit Mars to natal Moon quincunx is coming from a life giving house (5th sign from asc.), and therefore is not life threatening.

In my judgment, the grand trine of transit Mars-Moon to the natal Mars-Venus-ascendant conjunction trio would overpower the weaker worrisome quincunx of transit Mars to natal Moon. This exercise of my judgment is called "weighting". Yes, the astrologer must sometimes solve planetary conundrums with personal judgment calls and hope for the best.

What other aspects do we find? Transit Jupiter is near the descendant. Transit North Node moves through the 8th house (surgery), in Aries, sign of the face/eyes. These testimonies are generally positive for facial surgery. Emphasis, by transits is on the client's 2nd, 3rd, 5th and 9th signs from ascendant. This is far better than a 6th, 8th or 12th malefic house combination!

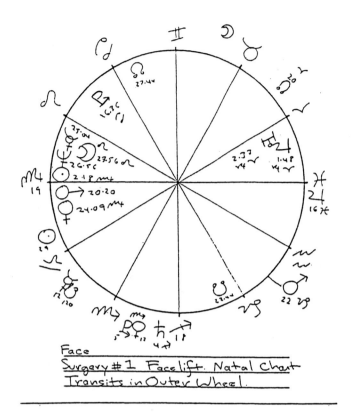

Face
Surgery #1 Facelift. Natal Chart
Transits in Outer Wheel.

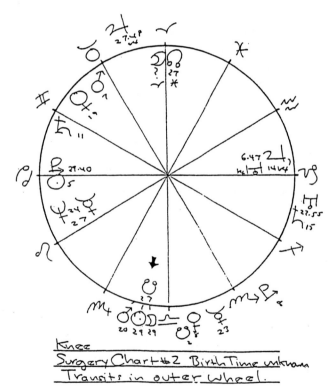

Knee
Surgery Chart #2 Birth Time unknown
Transits in outer Wheel.

SURGERY RESULTS FOR CHART #1

Scanning all client provided optional months for surgery parameters, I could find nothing that looked this good. The client, at first displeased with my choice of date, canceled vacation plans to use the suggested date. The surgery results were miraculous and well worth the exchange! My client's delicate skin healed without scarring in only two weeks and the surgeon could hardly believe it. There is no reason why your surgery elections cannot yield similarly wonderful results.

CHART #2: *Knee Replacement*
*Inner Wheel:* Natal solar chart.
*Outer wheel:* Transits for a knee replacement surgery that resulted in complications and death within two weeks.

CASE OVERVIEW

The patient's son contacted me about this already established surgery date. I adamantly suggested the abandonment or this date. Family was unwilling to shift to another, safer date. After all, they reasoned, knee replacement was a fairly routine procedure. What could possibly go wrong? The woman was never informed of my opinion, and surgery went ahead as planned: the replacement of the knee.

THE SURGERY CHART #2: *Knee Replacement*
*Discussion of chart and tactics.*

Does this woman have any planets in Capricorn, the sign of the knee? Or in Cancer, the opposite polarity to Capricorn? Yes - natal Jupiter, retrograde in Capricorn, angular; and Sun, Mercury and Neptune in opposite Cancer, angular. This combination reflects the knee trouble. We thus want it the Cancer-Capricorn well aspected by Mars, and fortified with good aspects. Remember our basic rule - ideally, transit Mars (the surgeons' knife) should be trine or sextile natal planets in Cancer-Capricorn. It is! So, what went wrong?

This should be a no-brainer for all you Lunar Node freaks.
• Transit Mars, Sun and a pre surgery eclipse are all conjunct the South Node, that big surgical "no-no".
• The eclipse, occurring only the previous day was conjunct her natal South Node by only one degree! Mars would reach the South Node, activating the eclipse effects within less than two weeks.
*continued*

• Transit Mercury is squaring its natal position. Transit Mercury is exactly
• Transit Venus quincunxes natal Mars.
• Transit Jupiter squares natal Mercury and is on the fatal nodal degrees.
• Transit Jupiter is in a sign that squares its natal position.
• Transit Jupiter squares natal Neptune.
• Transit Saturn opposes its natal position.
• Transit Neptune exactly opposes natal Sun from the descendant. (Because the descendant rules the doctors, Neptune's transit of this point warns of inattention, sloppy function or misdiagnosis on their part.)
• Transit Uranus quincunx to natal Neptune.
• Transit Pluto closely opposes natal Mars.
• Transit Neptune may square natal Moon (natal Moon sign unknown - either late Pisces or early Aries).
• Transit nodes square natal Sun - weakened anyway by the transit Neptune opposition. The Sun is therefore, in "the bends".

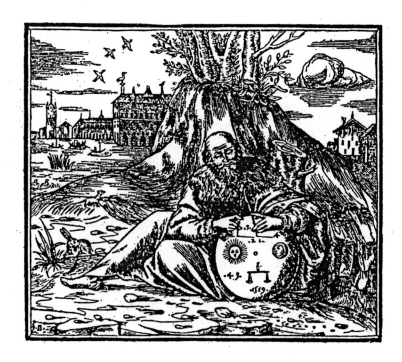

SURGERY RESULT FOR CHART #2:

Notice all those hard aspects both to natal Neptune and from transit Neptune? Neptune rules anesthesia. The transit Neptune opposite the Sun whilst the transit nodes square the Sun warn of a weakened heart (Sun) and danger through anesthesia (Neptune). The anesthesia went awry, resulting in a heart attack on the surgery table. The woman died within two weeks of the surgery.

This is perhaps the best example I've seen as to why we avoid those South Node transits. The South Node used to be called "the point of self undoing". Never, never, never time a surgery when Mars is near the South Node, even by sign for serious surgeries. This is my prime rule!


HOMEWORK FOR SERIOUS STUDENTS: Practice scanning your ephemeris for one year and finding all the dates when transit Mars is trine to any planet of your choice. Then, find a nearby date where the Moon is also sextile or trine the same planet. Can you get Mercury also in on the act, i.e., trining, or sextile the same planet? Is the natal South Node free of transits?

What of the other "don'ts" listed earlier in the preceding article? Don't get frustrated. It is next to impossible to find a perfect date as there is something always wrong somewhere. Work to know how to weight what is most essential in a mixed testimony set of transits. Learn to make decisions. Know what astrological conditions are unacceptable and acceptable. Soon, you will be good enough to help your clients have relatively complication free surgery dates.

# DO PLANETS ASPECT HOUSES?

Modern Western astrologers infrequently cite the concept of planetary aspects to the astrological houses of the birth chart. Saturn, Mars or Jupiter are not thought to cast rays upon houses, but only to each other and to the other planets.

The Vedic astrologers observe that planets do very much cast their rays upon the opposite house, and sometimes to the houses sextiling, squaring, trining and quincunxing their natal position. In their system, each planet has its own uniquely strongest aspects in relationship to the houses. For instance, Saturn is always considered to cast both a foreward sextile, and backwards square (according to the natural order of the signs); whereas Mars prefers the foreward square and quincunx. Jupiter's strongest aspect is the forward trine, and so forth.

Medical astrologers need concern themselves with what works and be willing to investigate what others have observed to be true. There will be cases where the obvious astrological source of a medical condition is an aspect to the house ruling the body part, rather than to the sign. Very serious conditions will be often be indicated in all possible ways.

For instance, a birth defect of the hand would be shown by an afflicted Mercury yes, and probably also afflictions to the mutable signs because the third and mutable sign Gemini rules the hand. However, you might find too, that natal Saturn is squaring the natal third house (associated with the hand); which also receives the quincunx from Mars, and an opposition from Neptune to boot! Thus we see the weak hand reflected by afflictions to the planet of the hand (Mercury); the sign of the hand (Gemini) and also the house of the hand (third house).

Be sure to consider the possibility that planets do cast their rays upon houses, influencing the form and function of the organs and body parts under their dominion.

# Epilogue

It is hoped that this generation will see a greater awareness of the influence of the Sun, Moon and planets upon the entire being of man and woman. Humankind has developed many new methods for peering ever deeper into the human organism and yet due to a cultural prejudice against astrology, we neglect the study of the lunar tides upon our very brain and bloodstreams!

Are we not more complex than Professor Brown's experimental oysters who opened with each overhead passage of the Moon, despite their removal to a new time zone far from the ocean's tide? Should not we too feel the Moon?

The effects of Sunlight, so profound, upon vegetation can not help but influence us in our own seasons of life.

And what of the known interference caused by planets upon radio transmission (Nelson, RCA)? Are not our very cells radio receivers in miniature? (Lakhovsky).

Let us envision a radical future, in which no surgery is undertaken without first consulting the positions of the planets in the birth chart of the patient! In such a world, no medicine would be taken under inappropriate Moon phases, as goes on today, and eclipses would be anathema for all but mandatory treatment.

Surgeons would consult their own charts for best and worst dates before scheduling their calendars. Children would be astrologically scanned for planetary health "signatures" and their parents provided with tailor made preventative programs. Hospitals would house a Department of Astral Medicine, staffed with superbly trained professionals.

Treatments given, and their timing, would be designed to suit you personally, based in part, upon your cosmobiological design.

No, embracing this ancient knowledge would not return us to a barbarous and ignorant past of bloodletting. Rather, we would reclaim the baby of wisdom tossed out with the bath water of ignorance when the scientific and industrial ages progressed.

May you who studies this wonderful subject contribute to this future time and bless those about you with the ageless gift of medical astrology.

*And Nature, the old Nurse, took*
*The child upon her knee,*
*Saying, "Here is a story book*
*Thy father hath written for thee".*

*"Come wander with me," she said,*
*"Into regions yet untrod,*
*And read what is still unread*
*In the manuscripts of God".*

*And he wandered away and away*
*With Nature, the dear old Nurse,*
*Who sang to him night and day*
*The rhymes of the universe.*     Longfellow

# Bibliography

*Christian Astrology*, William Lilly, Originally Published 1647, Regulus Publishing Co, Ltd., 1985, facsimile edition.

*The Tetrobiblios*, Claudius Ptolemy, Originally Published in 140 A.D., reprinted by Chicago Press, Illinois, 1936.

*Encyclopedia of Medical Astrology*, H.L. Cornell, M.D., Llewellyn Publications and Samuel Weiser, Inc., NYC, 1972.

*Medical Astrology*, Omar V. Garrison, Warner Paperback Library, 1973.

*The Healing Herbs of the Zodiac*, Ada Muir, Llewellyn Publications, 1974.

*The Astrology Guide to Good Health*, Alexandra Kayhle, Wilshire Book Company, 1968 edition.

*A Handbook of Medical Astrology*, Jane Ridder-Patrick, Arkana, Penguin Books, London and NY, 1990.

*Astrology, Nutrition and Health*, Robert Carl Jansky, Para Research, 1977.

*The Body Magnetic*, Buryl Payne, Ph.D., Copyright 1988.

*Astro-Diagnosis, A Guide to Healing*, Max Heindel, The Rosicrucian Fellowship, 7th edition, 1972, copyright 1929.

*Principals and Practice of Medical Astrology*, Dr. Jagannath Rao, Saggar Publications, New Delhi, 1972.

*Ptlolemy's Tetrabiblios*, Claudius Ptolemy, 140 A.D., reprinted, The Aries Press, Chicago,1936.

*Davidson's Medical Lectures*, A Series of Eight Special Lectures, Dr. William M. Davidson, The Astrological Bureau, Monroe, N.Y. (first taped 1959? printed 1979? unclear).

*Introduction to Medical Astrology*, Dr. William M. Davidson, The Astrological Bureau, Monroe, N. Y., Third Edition, 1978.

*Stellar Healing*, C.C. Zain, The Brotherhood of Light.

*Case Notes of a Medical Astrologer*, Margaret Millard, M.D., Samuel Weiser, NY, New York, 1980.

*The Healing Power of Gemstones*, Harish Johari, Destiny Books, Rochester, Vermont, 1988.

*Astrological Healing Gems*, Shivaji Bhattacharjee, Passage Press, Salt Lake City, UT, 1990.

*Gems and Astrology, A guide to health, happiness and prosperity*, Dr. Gouri Shanker Kapoor, Rajan Publications, New Delhi, 1985.

*The Metal-Planet Relationship*, Nick Kollerstrom, Borderland Sciences Research Foundation, Garberville, CA., 1993.

*Metal Magic*, Mellie Uyldert, Turnstone Press, Wellingborough, Northhamptonshire, 1980, (first published in Holland as *Wezen en Krachten der Metalen*, Amsterdam, 1980).

*The Astrological Body Types*, revised, Judith A. Hill, Borderland Research Sciences, Bayside, CA., 1997, all rights to Stellium Press, Portland, OR. Also available in Russian and Lettish editions through Astroinformserviss.

*The Arcana of Astrology*, W. J. Simmonite, New Castle Publishing Company, Inc., Newcastle Publishing Co., Inc., Van Nuys, CA. ISBN 0-87877-026-7.

*Degrees of the Zodiac*, Donna Walter Henson, A.F.A., Inc., 1981.

*The Astrology of Accidents*, C.E.O. Carter, Theological Publishing House Ltd., London, 1978.

*Astrology and the Edgar Cayce Readings*, Margaret H. Gammon, A.R.E. Press, Virginia Beach, Virginia, 1967.

*Electional Astrology*, Vivien E. Robson, Samuel Weiser, 1972.

*Dictionary of Astrology* by Fred Gettings, Routledge and Kegan Paul, London, 1985.

*Encyclopedia of Astrology*, Nicholas Devore, Philosophy Library of New York, Crown Books (no date given).

*The Mystery and Romance of Astrology*, C. J. S. Thompson, Causeway Books, 1973.

*A History of Western Astrology*, Jim Tester, Ballantine Books, 1989.

*The Geometry of Meaning*, Arthur Young, Robert Briggs and Associates, 1976.

*The Reflexive Universe*, Arthur Young, Robert Briggs and Associates.

*Twelve Signs, Twelve Sons*, David Womak.

*The Cosmic Clocks*, Michel Gauquelin, published with arrangement by Henry Regnery Company, 1969, Avon Books, New York, New York.

*Astrological Birth Control*, A Report on the Work of Dr. Eugen Jonas by Sheila Ostrander and Lynn Schroeder, Prentice Hall, N.J., 1972.

## JOURNAL ARTICLES

"Anatomical Correspondences to Zodiacal Degrees", translated by Mary L. Vohryzek, appearing in "NCGR Journal", Medical Edition, 1985, translated by Mary L. Vohryzek from Elsbeth and Reinhold Ebertin's *Anatomische Entsprechungen der Tierkreisgrade*.

## ADDITIONAL READING

*Alternative Complementary Health Compendium: Astrological Judgment of Diseases From the Decumbiture of the Sick*, Nicholas Culpeper

*Astrological Healing*, Reinhold Ebertin

*Astrology of Childbirth*, Doris Chase Doane

*Culpeper's Complete Herbal* (17th century)

*Healing with Astrology*, Marcia Starck

*Healing with the Horoscope*, Maritha Pottenger

*Medical Astrology* -Ingrid Naiman
Volume 1: Stress; Volume 2: The Elements
Volume 3: Astro-endocrinology; Volume 4: Cancer

*Essentials of Medical Astrology*, K.S. Charak
*Medical Astrology*, Heinrish Daath

*Planetary Influences and Therapeutic Uses of Precious Stones* - G. Kunz

*How to Give an Astrological Health Reading*, Diane Cramer M.S.

## MORE BOOKS BY JUDITH A. HILL
### Available from Stellium Press

*The Astrological Body Types*, revised and expanded, Stellium Press, 1997, (available through New Leaf, A.F. A. Inc., Stellium Press).

*Vocational Astrology*, A.F.A. Inc., 1999 (winner of the A.F.A. Inc., Paul R. Grell "Best Book" Award for A.F.A. books, 1999). Also available from A.F.A.

*The Part of Fortune in Astrology*, Stellium Press, 1998.

*The Mars-Redhead Files*, Stellium Press, 2000.

*Astroseismology: Earthquakes and Astrology*, Stellium Press, 2000.

*Tales From Hedgehog Crossing*, Stellium Press, 2003.

JOURNAL ARTICLES BY JUDITH A. HILL

Judith A. Hill & Jacalyn Thompson, "The Mars–Redhead Link", *NCGR Journal*, Winter 88-89 (Also published by *Above & Below*, Canada, first publication; *Linguace Astrale* (Italy); *AA Journal* (Great Britain); *FAA Journal* (Australia).

"The Mars Redhead Link II: Mars Distribution Patterns in Redhead Populations", *Borderlands Research Sciences Foundation Journal*, Vol. L1, No. 1 (part one) and Vol. L1, No 2 (part 2).

"Commentary on the John Addey Redhead Data", *NCGR Journal*, Winter 88-89.

"Redheads and Mars", (the replication research) *The Mountain Astrologer*, May 1996.

"The Regional Factor in Planetary-Seismic Correlation", *Borderlands Research Sciences Foundation Journal*, Vol. L1, Number 3, 1995 (reprint courtesy of *American Astrology*).

Judith A. Hill & Mark Polit, "Correlation of Earthquakes with Planetary Placement: The Regional Factor", *NCGR Journal*, 5 (1), 1987.

"American Redhead's Project Replication", *Correlation*, Volume 13, No 2, Winter 94-95.

"Octaves of Time", *Borderlands Research Journal*, Vol. L1, Number 4, Fourth Quarter, 1995.

"Gemstones, Antidotes for Planetary Weaknesses", *ISIS Journal*, *1994.*

"Medical Astrology", *Borderlands Research Journal*, Vol. L11, Number 1, First Quarter, 1996.

"Astrological Heredity", *Borderlands Research Journal*, 1996.

"The Electional and Horary Branches", *Sufism, IAS*, Vol. 1, No 2

"Astrology: A Philosophy of Time and Space", *Sufism, IAS*, Vol. 1, No 1

"Natal Astrology", *Sufism, IAS*, Vol. 1, No 3

"An Overview of Medical Astrology", *Sufism, IAS*, Vol. 1, No 4

"Predictive Astrology in Theory and Practice", *Sufism, IAS*, Vol. 11, No 1

"Esoteric Astrology", *Sufism, IAS*, Vol. 11, No 2, 3

"Mundane Astrology", *Sufism, IAS*, Vol. 11, No 4

"Vocational Astrology", *Sufism, IAS*, part 1 and 2, Vol. 111, No 1, 2

"Astro-Psychology", Vol. 111, No 3, 4

"The Planetary Time Clocks", *Sufism, IAS*, Vol. 4, No 1, 2, 3, 4

"Astrophysiognomy", *Sufism, IAS*, Vol. 4, No 1, 2

"Spiritual Signposts in the Birth Map", *Sufism, IAS*, Vol. V, No 2, 3

"The Philosophical Questions Most Frequently Asked of the Astrologer", *Sufism, IAS*, Vol. 5, No 4, Vol. 6, No 1, 2

"Music and the Ear of the Beholder", *Sufism*, IAS, 1999.

"The Astrology of Diabetes", *Dell Horoscope*, October 2003.

## Biography of Author

Judith Hill is a lifetime astrological consultant who has accomplished many thousands of astrological readings. She has served as the Educational Director for the San Francisco National Council for Geocosmic Research and as a faculty member for The Institute of Stellar Influence Studies. She holds the degree of *Chartered Herbalist* with the Dominion College of Herbal Sciences.

Ms. Hill achieved 100% accuracy in the matching of five anonymous birth charts to biographies in a 1986 skeptic designed NCGR sponsored challenge.

She is the author of six books including the classic *The Astrological Body Types*. Judith received the Paul R. Grell *Best Book Award* for A.F.A. Inc. Books published in 1999-2000 for her *Vocational Astrology: A Complete Handbook of Western Astrological Career Selection and Guidance Techniques*.

Her works enjoy an international audience and her books and writings have been translated into several languages including Russian, Lettish, and Italian.

Hill's scientific research on the subjects of astrogenetics and astroseismology are world renowned. She was partner in the Hill-Polit breakthrough seismic research of the 1980s, and was awarded a research grant from the Institute for the Study of Consciousness.

Hill was the founder of Redheads Research, an internationally acclaimed project of ten years duration, conducted with Jacalyn Thompson, investigating the position of Mars in the charts of redheaded people.

Judith has made numerous TV and radio appearances and lectures widely on a wide range of fascinating metaphysical topics.

She can be contacted by email at stelliumpress@aol.com